Low Sodium, Big Flavor

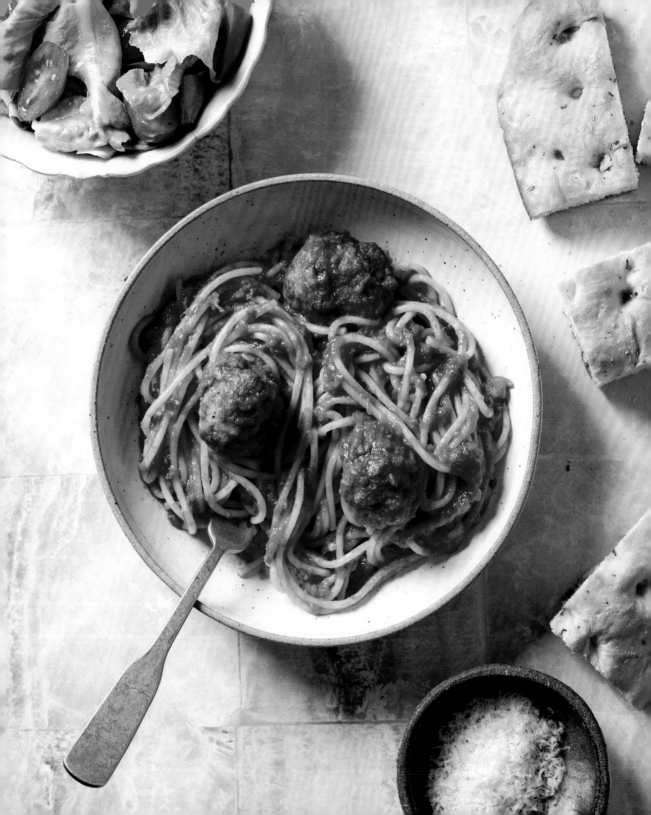

Low Sodium, Big Flavor

115 Recipes for Pantry Staples and Daily Meals

Lara Ferroni

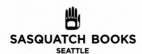

SASQUATCH BOOKS

SEATTLE

Printed in China

SASQUATCH BOOKS with colophon is a registered trademark of Penguin Random House LLC

25 24 23 22 21   9 8 7 6 5 4 3 2 1

Editor: Susan Roxborough
Production editor: Rachelle Longé McGhee
Photography and styling: Lara Ferroni
Designer: Tony Ong

Library of Congress Cataloging-in-Publication Data
Name: Ferroni, Lara, author.
Title: Low sodium, big flavor : 115 Recipes for Pantry Staples and Daily Meals / Lara Ferroni.
Description: Seattle : Sasquatch Books, [2021] | Includes index.
Identifiers: LCCN 2020019643 (print) | LCCN 2020019644 (ebook) | ISBN 9781632172860 (paperback) | ISBN 9781632172877 (ebook)
Subjects: LCSH: Salt-free diet--Recipes. | LCGFT: Cookbooks.
Classification: LCC RM237.8 .F47 2021 (print) | LCC RM237.8 (ebook) | DDC 641.5/6323--dc23
LC record available at https://lccn.loc.gov/2020019643
LC ebook record available at https://lccn.loc.gov/2020019644

ISBN: 978-1-63217-286-0

Sasquatch Books
1904 Third Avenue, Suite 710
Seattle, WA 98101
SasquatchBooks.com

Contents

MAINS

SIDES

DESSERTS

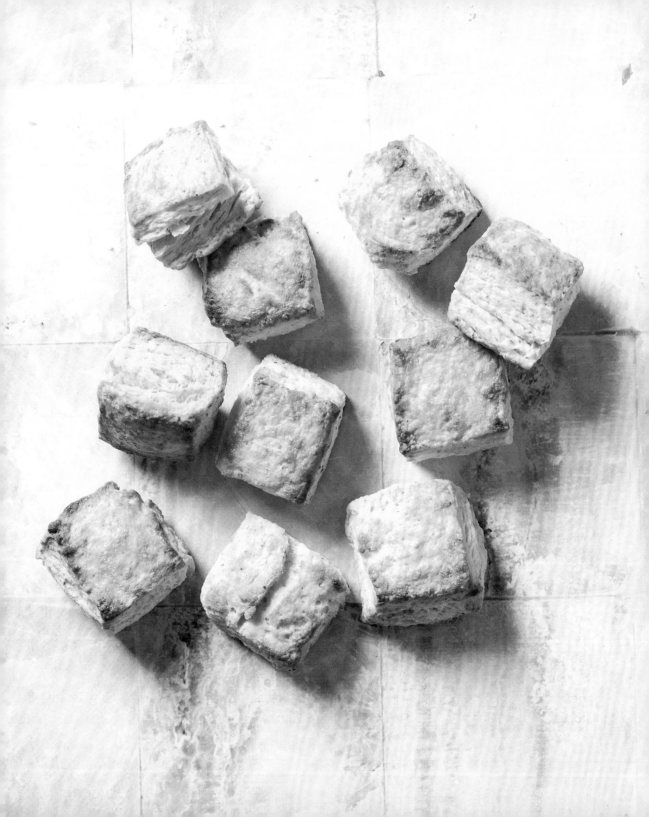

Introduction

Several years ago, I was diagnosed with Ménière's disease, a syndrome most known for a combination of hearing loss and drop attacks (sudden vertigo where the world goes topsy-turvy). My diagnosis came after two years of intermittent hearing loss and tinnitus in one ear. So far, I'm one of the lucky ones who hasn't had any drop attacks (yes, that's wood you hear me knocking on). Still, my balance is not what it used to be, and I have associated BPPV (benign paroxysmal positional vertigo) attacks, along with some serious brain fog during my episodes.

The good news is that, while it can be incredibly debilitating, Ménière's isn't fatal. Many sufferers can control it with diet and lifestyle changes: eliminating caffeine, cutting back significantly on alcohol, and keeping daily sodium to 1,500 milligrams or less.

I'm a food writer, recipe developer, and photographer, and I really love to eat good food. Until my diagnosis, I always had the luxury of consuming what I wanted without having to think about it. Now I had to make changes, and my first thought was, What the @#!%$ am I going to eat?

I realized I had no idea how much sodium was in my food, so I did what most people do: I googled. My first question was, How much sodium is in a teaspoon of salt? Google's answer didn't make me happy. In turns out that a single teaspoon of table salt contains 2,325 milligrams of sodium—30 percent more than I was aiming to consume in a day! Doesn't every recipe call for about a teaspoon of salt? OK, I reasoned, I can just cut way down on the salt in recipes. That should do it, right?

Unfortunately, there are all sorts of sneaky sodium sources that I never even realized. While the recommended daily sodium allowance for a healthy person is 2,500 milligrams, I've come to seriously doubt that most people consume anywhere near that number. Just one slice of cheese pizza contains about 1,500 milligrams. A plain bagel has 400. That blueberry muffin that doesn't taste salty at all? It probably has about 500 milligrams, thanks to the baking powder in it. Heck, a few cups of kale contains 50 milligrams, and even celery, which is like eating crunchy air, has 32 milligrams per stalk. My guess is that I was previously consuming 4,000 to 6,000 milligrams a day.

The first time I went grocery shopping after committing to a reduced-sodium diet, I found myself standing in the aisle, in shock, thinking I'd never be able to eat anything good again. Everything I picked up seemed to have more sodium than I expected. Trying to figure out what I could eat was overwhelming. I managed to pick up a few random things and made myself a dinner that tasted like . . . well, like it needed salt.

I spent about a week wallowing in self-pity, painstakingly monitoring my sodium intake. On most days I kept it to under 1,000 milligrams by mostly eating super-plain food. I ate a lot of oatmeal that first week. Lots and lots of oatmeal.

But it got better. Slowly, as I learned how to amp up flavor with spices and acids, and my palate adjusted, eating started to become a joy again and not (for the most part) a stress-induced nightmare.

In this book I share my low-sodium cooking techniques, tips, and recipes for anyone who needs to manage their sodium. News flash: I'm not a doctor, and I'm not a nutritionist. Be sure to consult your doctor regarding recommended nutritional requirements.

Each recipe in this book provides a total sodium count and, where it makes sense, a per-serving sodium amount. Note that optional ingredients are factored into the total. To calculate the sodium in a recipe, I used information from ingredient labels or reliable sources that I trust, such as the Food and Drug Administration, the US Department of Agriculture, and the UK Department of Health and Social Care. For recipes such as the fresh cheeses (pages 105 to 109), where sodium can't accurately be calculated from the ingredients, I used a sodium ion meter to measure the sodium count. That said, the ingredients you purchase may have different sodium levels than mine. Where it makes sense, I list specific brands, or alert you to brands that contain less sodium. I urge you to read labels carefully for sodium levels.

In the first section, I include recipes for low-sodium versions of pantry staples that you probably currently buy premade, such as condiments, soup stocks, and breads. These recipes may take a bit more time and energy, but the effort is well worth it because they save you both sodium and money.

In the second section, you'll find recipes for daily dishes, so you have lots of options for breakfast, lunch, and dinner. They are easily paired with other recipes for complete low-sodium meals, and most make use of the low-sodium sauces, condiments, and spice mixes in the book as well. Because having time to cook—especially if you are also making your own pantry staples—is a luxury, most of the recipes are designed to come together quickly, with options for one-pot mains and yields that give you leftovers for even quicker serving later.

You can also visit my website LowSodiumBigFlavor.com for more tools to help you manage your daily intake. There you'll find meal-plan suggestions that make it easy to keep within a 1,200 to 1,800 milligram daily range. I also provide a searchable database of approximate sodium counts for common foods that goes beyond the Sodium Counts for Common Ingredients table on page 243. Knowing your ingredients will help you make smart substitutions in the recipes you already love to cook, or those you want to try.

I hope you enjoy the recipes in this book as much as I do, and that they bring a new variety of meals to your dinner table. Most importantly, my goal is that once you've gotten the hang of how and when to substitute ingredients and enhance flavor without salt, you'll be comfortable adapting recipes from any cookbook or website.

Before You Begin

Getting started with a low-sodium diet may mean you will be cooking more than you used to, so set up your kitchen for success with my recommended tools and pantry ingredients. A few of the spices that I have in my kitchen may not be readily available in your local grocery store, but there are great online sources, such as World Spice Merchants (WorldSpice.com), The Spice House (TheSpiceHouse.com), Penzey's (Penzeys.com), and Amazon.com.

¶

KITCHEN TOOLS

What follows is a partial list of the tools I use in my kitchen (a complete list would take an entire book in itself—I tend to go a little overboard in the kitchen-tool department). You'll definitely want the basics: a good sharp knife, spatulas, skillets, measuring cups, and the like, but there are also a few pieces of equipment you may not currently have that I use frequently to make these recipes.

Baking Pans
I have a lot of baking pans: half-sheet pans (13 by 18 inches), quarter-sheet pans (9 by 13 inches), muffin tins (with 2-by-1¼-inch cups), pie pans (9 inch), cake pans (8 inch and 9 inch), and a fluted tube pan (also known as a Bundt pan). While you can make do in a pinch, the right pan is important for getting the right results.

Pan size is particularly essential for yeast-based pan-loaf breads, in order to get the right shape. The yeast-bread recipes in this book (such as Honey Whole Wheat Sandwich Bread on page 43) make two loaves and use 8½-by-4½-by-3-inch loaf pans. If your loaves turn out too flat, your pans may be too big.

Blender (Countertop or Immersion)

I use my countertop blender a lot. I have a Vitamix, but any brand will work for the recipes in this book, which do not contain anything too hard that would require a heavy-duty blender.

An immersion blender, also called a hand or stick blender, is very useful for making salad dressings and other small-quantity sauces that would be hard for a countertop blender to handle. A stick blender also takes the work out of making homemade mayonnaise. If you are purchasing one for the first time, consider choosing one that comes with accessories such as a whisk attachment and a small chopper, which can replace a food processor for many recipes.

Dutch Oven

An enameled Dutch oven is great for slow roasting, baking your own rustic bread, or even for deep-frying. Lodge makes fantastic versions in a variety of colors and sizes at very reasonable prices. I use my 4-quart Dutch oven all the time.

Food Processor

While it's not a requirement, a food processor will really speed up and simplify your food prep. Ideally, your food processor will also have an insert to quickly pulverize smaller amounts that the full-size work bowl may not handle well, such as grinding ½ cup of spices to make a blend.

Heating Pad

Yep, the kind you use for a sore back also makes an excellent pad for rising yeast doughs if the room is a little cold. I set mine on the lowest temperature and place it on top of the bowl the dough is rising in.

Multicooker/Pressure Cooker

A multicooker, such as the Instant Pot, combines the functionality of a pressure cooker, slow cooker, and rice cooker into a single appliance that becomes pretty indispensable once you get used to cooking with it. Just the ability to cook dried beans (since canned beans are loaded with sodium) in forty minutes instead of four hours (plus soaking time!) is worth it to me, even if I didn't use my Instant Pot for other purposes all the time. It's also great when you want some comfort food, but don't have the energy for cooking. There are lots of dishes that only require you to throw all the ingredients into the pot and turn it on—and 40 minutes later, dinner is ready. I use a 6-quart Instant Pot DUO60.

If a multicooker isn't in your budget, a simple stovetop pressure cooker can often be found for less than $30 new, and most recipes that call for a multicooker are using the pressure-cooker feature.

Stand Mixer

If you make your own baked goods, a stand mixer with paddle and dough hook attachments is a real boon. It may take a little more work than a bread machine, but you'll use it for more than just bread, so I think it's the better choice if you have limited space. I recommend getting at least a 5-quart mixer with a 325-watt motor. However, I can make all the baked goods in this book with a KitchenAid 3.5-quart mixer with a 250-watt motor (the KitchenAid Artisan Mini). I have to stop and start the mixer a few extra times when making larger batches of dough, but it gets the job done.

PANTRY INGREDIENTS

Amchoor Powder

Amchoor powder (sometimes spelled *amchur* or *amhur*) is made from dried, unripe mangoes and adds a buttery tartness that can be a great salt replacement in some recipes. It's one of the key ingredients in my Popcorn Seasoning (page 33). You can find *amchoor* powder at some Asian grocers, or online at The Spice House, World Spice Merchants, or Amazon.

Aquafaba

Aquafaba is the liquid in canned beans; some crazy sorcery makes it act like eggs in recipes, especially those that call for whipped egg whites. Although you can use the water from any type of bean, chickpea liquid is preferred for its mild taste. Of course, canned chickpea water is a no-no for those on a low-sodium diet, but you can make your own sodium-free version by rehydrating dried chickpeas.

You may be wondering why you should bother. Eggs have a reasonable amount of sodium—about 70 milligrams per egg. For most recipes, it's not enough for me to worry about. But if you are really trying to trim your sodium, or if a recipe calls for a lot of eggs, aquafaba can be a nice substitute. A good rule of thumb is that 3 tablespoons of aquafaba replaces one whole egg.

Chili Flakes

My pantry is full of chili flakes. I'm endlessly intrigued by any variety I stumble upon. The traditional red pepper flakes, the ones you shake onto your pizza, are typically made from cayenne peppers, or a mix that is mostly cayenne. I've got a tinful of flakes that I generously sprinkle on just about anything. I also have jars of Aleppo pepper flakes, Korean *gochugaru* flakes, and chipotle flakes, which have varying levels of heat, fruitiness, and smokiness. I encourage you to try a few options and find the chilies that work for you. World Spice Merchants is a great source for a wide selection of chili flakes that you might not find in your regular market.

Citric Acid

Also called citric salt or sour salt, citric acid powder is used in some cheese-making to separate out the curds, but a pinch also adds a bit of tartness to recipes, such as my Lemon Pepper (page 36). You may not find citric acid in your grocery store, but it's easily available online.

Coconut Aminos

Coconut aminos is a gluten-free, lower sodium soy sauce substitute made from fermented coconut palm sap. It has a mild salty sweetness that blends well with savory and smoky flavors. It's not low in sodium, but it has 90 milligrams per teaspoon instead of the 280 milligrams in regular soy sauce. The amount of sodium in coconut aminos is similar to low-sodium soy sauce, but I prefer its more complex flavor.

Dried Pasta

Dried pasta is a bit of a miracle to me. My homemade pasta contains salt, so I assumed that the regular store-bought dried stuff would too. But what a pleasant surprise! It almost always has zero sodium (though do check the label anyway, as some brands may add it).

Light Salt

Typically a mixture of iodized salt and potassium chloride, low-sodium salt has about 1,100 milligrams per teaspoon, or roughly half the sodium of fine-grain salt, with not much difference in flavor. Light salt is only available as fine grain, so it isn't a great substitute for flaky or coarse finishing salt in terms of texture, but a pinch sprinkled on as a garnish can provide the same salty bite. I use Morton Lite Salt (available in many large grocery stores, as well as online) for cooking and baking, usually reducing the quantity in a standard recipe by about half. There is also a version of sodium-free salt substitute that is entirely potassium chloride, but it has an aftertaste. Note that if you're watching your potassium intake, you may want to be careful with this.

Low-Sodium Cheeses

Most cheese is very high in sodium and therefore best avoided. However, both Swiss cheese and fresh mozzarella are on the lower end of the sodium spectrum, so they are great choices when you have a craving.

Paprika

Paprika, made from finely ground dried red peppers, isn't really a replacement for salt, but it does add a lot of flavor to dishes, so you'll forget that you miss the salt. Paprika comes in many forms: smoked or unsmoked, hot or mild (sometimes called sweet), Spanish or Hungarian. Also, if you can find it, piment d'Espelette is a more coarsely ground red chili pepper with a fruity, bold flavor. Keep a few different types on hand to create the right taste for whatever dish you are cooking.

Peppercorns

Peppercorns will become one of your new best friends for adding flavor to food. Avoid preground pepper, which has a fraction of the flavor of freshly ground. And there's no need to stick to just black peppercorns; try red, green, and white versions, as well as Tellicherry, which are larger black peppercorns with a complex floral, earthy flavor. World Spice Merchants carries a great selection, including a smoked black pepper. A tip: The little prefilled plastic pepper grinders are inexpensive and refillable, so once you've used the peppercorns in them (I recommend the mixed blend), you can replenish them with any peppercorns you'd like.

Shichimi Togarashi

Togarashi is the Japanese word for chilies, although the spice mix, typically called *shichimi togarashi*, or seven spice, contains a blend of seasonings, which usually include nori (seaweed), orange peel, sesame seeds, poppy seeds, and garlic—but luckily, no salt! (However, do check the label, just in case.) While there is some sodium in the nori, the spice mix overall is low in sodium.

Sodium-Free Baking Powder

There are multiple brands with different mixtures for sodium-free baking powder, but the one I find works best is Hain Pure Foods Featherweight Baking Powder, which contains a combination of potassium bicarbonate, monocalcium phosphate, and potato starch. It's available online and in many large grocery stores. It's designed to be used measure-for-measure in baking recipes, but for best results I usually use a "heaping" measure when I'm substituting it for regular baking powder.

Sodium-Free Baking Soda

Sodium-free baking soda is typically made from a combination of calcium carbonate and magnesium carbonate, so it's free of both potassium and sodium. It's considerably weaker than regular baking soda (sodium bicarbonate), so you'll need to double up on the quantity called for in a typical recipe. (However, the recipes in this book are specifically designed for sodium-free baking soda, so don't double it in these!) I use Ener-G Baking Soda Substitute, which you can purchase online.

Sumac

Sumac is made from the ground, dried berries of a native Middle Eastern bush and adds a bright, lemony flavor—as well as a lovely deep-red color—to any dish. It's great in rubs for meat or just sprinkled on as a garnish. Cooking sumac somewhat dulls its flavor, so don't shy away from using larger quantities in cooked dishes. When you purchase it, make sure it only contains ground sumac berries; some sumac is sold with added salt.

Unsalted Canned Tomatoes

Most canned tomatoes contain quite a bit of salt, but at well-stocked grocery stores you can usually find no-salt-added versions, which have 25 milligrams or less per ½ cup. I like Pomì brand strained tomato sauce and chopped tomatoes, Muir Glen whole tomatoes, and Amore tomato paste.

Vinegar/Citrus

Acid is a critical flavor component; without it, food tastes bland or flat. Salt provides the acid in most recipes, but using a different acid can work to brighten the flavor.

I add lemon juice or lemon zest to many recipes to perk them up, so I try to keep a bowl of fresh lemons around at all times. Bottled lemon juice works too; I prefer the kind not made from concentrate.

Vinegar is another key ingredient in my pantry. I keep several different kinds: red wine, sherry, apple cider, and balsamic vinegars are my staples. The quality makes a huge difference in the flavor, so it's worth splurging on at least a couple of good bottles. For example, Katz Late Harvest Zinfandel vinegar (KatzFarm.com) is a zingy, jammy red wine vinegar that brings the wow to any salad (I could pretty much drink it by the spoonful).

White vinegars are virtually sodium-free. Red vinegars have a tiny bit of sodium, which varies by type, but it's still negligible. Look for rice vinegar (also called rice wine vinegar) that's labeled unseasoned, as seasoned rice vinegar contains salt and sugar.

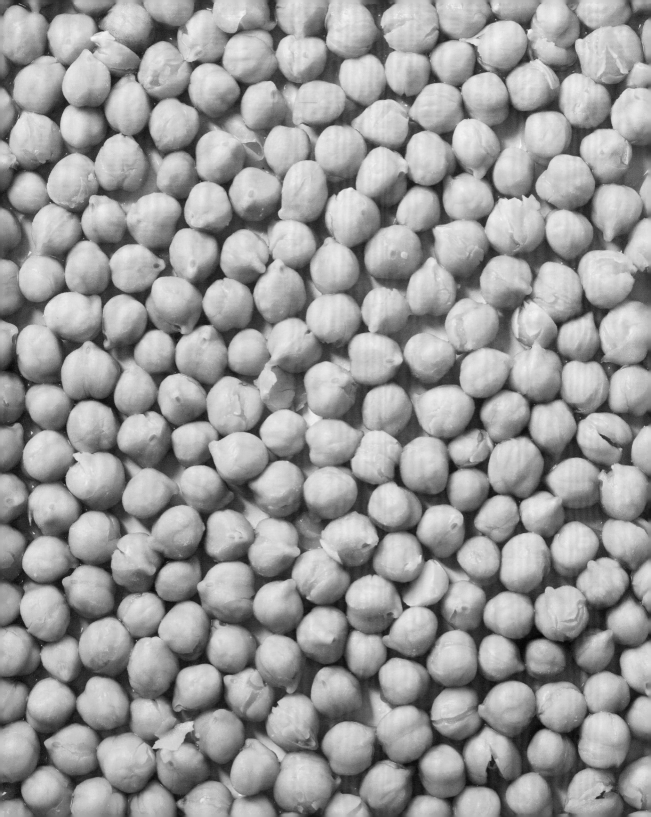

PART I:

STAPLES

Just leaving out the salt when you cook, or at the dinner table, isn't enough if the ingredients you use are high in sodium. Sodium lurks in all sorts of prepared foods: baked goods, condiments, cheeses, salad dressings, and processed meats are the main offenders. Luckily, there's no need to cut these foods out of your life entirely. With a little bit of planning and elbow grease in the kitchen, there are low-sodium alternatives you can make—and they may even reduce your food budget!

Many of the recipes in this section—including most of the condiments and many of the baked goods—can be made ahead of time and kept in your pantry or freezer, so they are just as convenient as those purchased premade.

Condiments

Ketchup

Most of the time when I try fancy "house-made" ketchup, I'm disappointed. Like many of us, I equate ketchup with Heinz and view anything else as an entirely different food—even if it tastes good, it's just not right. Unfortunately, Heinz ketchup has 160 milligrams of sodium per tablespoon. So, while it may be fine to dip the odd french fry in, it's pretty much off the acceptable list.

I don't promise that this ketchup will taste exactly like Heinz. In fact, it won't, because it has only a fraction of the salt. But it does have a close balance of acid to sweet to spice. And I think you'll like it.

Makes: About 2 cups
TOTAL SODIUM: 565 mg
SODIUM PER TABLESPOON:
  About 18 mg

2 tablespoons olive oil
1 cup chopped onion
1 clove garlic, chopped
2 cups tomato puree

¼ cup lightly packed light brown sugar
1 tablespoon light corn syrup
½ cup distilled white vinegar
1 tablespoon tomato paste
½ teaspoon light salt

⅛ teaspoon dry mustard
⅛ teaspoon ground cloves
⅛ teaspoon ground allspice
⅛ teaspoon cayenne pepper
⅛ teaspoon freshly ground black pepper

1   Heat the oil in a medium saucepan over medium heat. Add the onion and garlic and cook until the onions have softened and are translucent, about 5 minutes. Add the remaining ingredients and stir well to combine. Bring the mixture to a boil, reduce the heat to low, and simmer, stirring occasionally to avoid scorching, until the ketchup is thick enough to coat a spoon, 45 to 60 minutes.

2   Transfer the ketchup to a blender, observing precautions for hot liquids (fill it less than halfway, remove the blender lid's center insert, and hold a kitchen towel over the top), or to the bowl of a food processor and puree until smooth.

3   Store in an airtight container in the refrigerator for up to 1 month.

Mustard

Think of this recipe as a rough guide for you to customize. Yellow mustard seeds will produce the mildest mustard, while brown seeds are more pungent. I like a mix of the two, which makes a mustard similar to Dijon.

Makes: 1 cup

TOTAL SODIUM: 253 mg

SODIUM PER TABLESPOON:
About 17 mg

½ cup yellow or brown mustard seeds

¾ cup apple cider vinegar

⅔ cup water, divided

1¼ teaspoons granulated sugar

¼ teaspoon light salt

¼ teaspoon ground turmeric (optional)

1   Put the mustard seeds in a small bowl with the vinegar and ⅓ cup of the water, and soak them for 2 days.

2   After 2 days, stir in the sugar, salt, turmeric, and the remaining ⅓ cup water. For a smooth mustard: Puree the mixture in a blender or food processor until smooth, adding a little more vinegar or water if it gets too thick. Push it through a fine-mesh sieve for an even smoother mustard. For a whole grain mustard: Pulse the mixture in a food processor until the seeds are lightly crushed.

3   Store in an airtight container in the refrigerator for up to 6 months.

Mayonnaise

Store-bought mayonnaise contains about 90 milligrams of salt per tablespoon, compared to this low-sodium (but still plenty flavorful!) version's 22 milligrams. Your sandwiches will no longer have to go without.

You can make this in a food processor, but using an immersion blender lets you skip the finicky step of slowly streaming in the oil, which makes it a lot easier to prepare.

Makes: About ¾ cup

TOTAL SODIUM: 264 mg

SODIUM PER TABLESPOON:
About 22 mg

1 large egg yolk
¾ cup sunflower oil
1½ teaspoons freshly
  squeezed lemon juice

1 teaspoon white wine
  vinegar
¼ teaspoon light salt
Pinch of dry mustard

1   If you are using an immersion blender, in a tall jar that is just wide enough to fit the blender, layer the egg yolk, oil, juice, vinegar, salt, and mustard. Insert the blender all the way to the bottom of the jar, and puree for about 10 seconds on high without moving the blender. Then slowly move it up and down until the mayonnaise is completely blended.

2   If you are using a food processor, put the egg yolk, juice, vinegar, salt, and mustard in the bowl of the processor and pulse to combine. Then, while the processor is running, very slowly stream in the oil until the mayonnaise is completely blended. This should take a few minutes.

3   Store in an airtight container in the refrigerator for up to 1 week.

Louisiana-Style Hot Sauce

Check your local farmers' market from mid- to late summer for fresh cayenne peppers. You can also use whole dried cayenne peppers, which can be purchased online. Just rehydrate them first by soaking them in warm water for about ten minutes.

Makes: About 1 cup

TOTAL SODIUM: 570 mg
SODIUM PER TABLESPOON:
 About 36 mg

12 cayenne peppers or other hot red chili peppers, stemmed

1 cup distilled white vinegar
½ teaspoon light salt

1   In a small saucepan over medium-high heat, combine the peppers, vinegar, and salt. Bring to a boil, reduce the heat to medium-low, cover, and simmer for 20 minutes.

2   Transfer the mixture to a blender, observing precautions for hot liquids (fill it less than halfway, remove the blender lid's center insert, and hold a kitchen towel over the top), or to the bowl of a food processor and puree until smooth. Strain it through a fine-mesh sieve.

3   Store in an airtight bottle or jar in the refrigerator for up to 1 month.

Sriracha

Most sriracha recipes are fermented. Unfortunately, safely fermenting requires a relatively large amount of salt. This recipe skips the longer fermentation period (and all that sodium), yielding a lovely fresh alternative to the traditional "rooster sauce." Can't find red chilies? Just use green ones—your sriracha will be green, but taste just as delicious.

Makes: About 1 cup
TOTAL SODIUM: 515 mg
SODIUM PER TABLESPOON:
   About 32 mg

½ cup distilled white or white wine vinegar
½ teaspoon light salt
2 cloves garlic

½ pound hot red chili peppers, such as red Fresno or jalapeño
1 tablespoon lightly packed light brown sugar

1 In a small saucepan over medium-low heat, combine the vinegar, salt, and garlic. Stir until the salt has completely dissolved, about 1 minute, then take the pan off the heat and set aside.

2 Remove the stems from the chilies. If you want a less spicy sauce, also remove the seeds. Roughly chop the chilies, place them in a clean pint jar, and pour the vinegar mixture over the top. Cover, and let sit 8 to 20 hours.

3 Drain the mixture in a colander set over a bowl to preserve the brine. Put the chilies in a small pot over medium heat, stir in the sugar, and simmer for about 2 minutes, until the sugar has completely dissolved.

4 Transfer the chilies to a blender or food processor, and pulse until almost pureed. Add the brine ¼ cup at a time, pulsing after each addition until the mixture is smooth. You may not need to use all the brine.

5 Strain the sriracha through a fine-mesh sieve, using the back of a spoon to gently push it through the strainer to remove any seeds and skins.

6 Store in an airtight bottle or jar in the refrigerator for up to 1 month.

Harissa

Harissa is a North African hot chili paste made from a combination of dried red chilies and spices such as caraway and cumin, along with a healthy squeeze of citrus. There are many different varieties of harissa, some containing upwards of forty spices.

Makes: About 1 cup
TOTAL SODIUM: 571 mg
SODIUM PER TABLESPOON:
About 36 mg

1 cup water
4 dried guajillo chilies,
stemmed and seeded

4 dried ancho chilies,
stemmed and seeded
4 dried arbol chilies,
stemmed and seeded
2 teaspoons caraway
seeds
2 teaspoons coriander
seeds

1 teaspoon cumin seeds
3 cloves garlic, smashed
1 teaspoon smoked
paprika
½ teaspoon light salt
2 tablespoons olive oil
2 tablespoons freshly
squeezed lemon juice

1   Boil the water in a small saucepan over medium-low heat. Put the chilies in a large heatproof bowl. Pour the boiling water over the chilies and let them sit for 20 minutes to rehydrate them.

2   Meanwhile, in a small skillet over medium heat, toast the caraway, coriander, and cumin seeds until they are fragrant and popping, about 3 minutes. Transfer the seeds to the bowl of a food processor, add the garlic and 1 tablespoon of the water from the chilies, and pulse until most of the garlic is chopped, scraping down the sides of the bowl as needed.

3   Once the chilies have rehydrated, use a slotted spoon to remove them from the water (reserve the water) and add them, along with the paprika and salt, to the garlic mixture. Pulse until the chilies have formed a rough paste. If the mixture is too thick to puree, add more of the reserved chili water.

4   Add the olive oil and lemon juice, and pulse to combine.

5   Store in an airtight bottle or jar in the refrigerator for up to 1 month.

Barbecue Sauce

Homemade barbecue sauce is well worth making, even if you aren't doing it to cut down on sodium. It's easy; you can customize it to your preferred level of spice, sweetness, and tang; and it keeps well, so you can have it on hand for a quick grill or broil.

Makes: About 1½ cups

TOTAL SODIUM: 113 mg

SODIUM PER TABLESPOON:
   About 5 mg

———

1½ cups apple cider vinegar
½ cup lightly packed light brown sugar

½ cup tomato puree
¼ cup tomato paste
1 teaspoon coconut aminos
1 teaspoon smoked paprika

1 teaspoon freshly ground black pepper
½ teaspoon garlic powder
½ teaspoon dry mustard
½ teaspoon cayenne pepper (optional)

1   Combine all ingredients in a medium saucepan and simmer over medium-high heat for about 30 minutes, stirring frequently and scraping down the sides as needed, until the sauce thickens and reduces to about 1½ cups.

2   Store in an airtight bottle or jar in the refrigerator for up to 1 month.

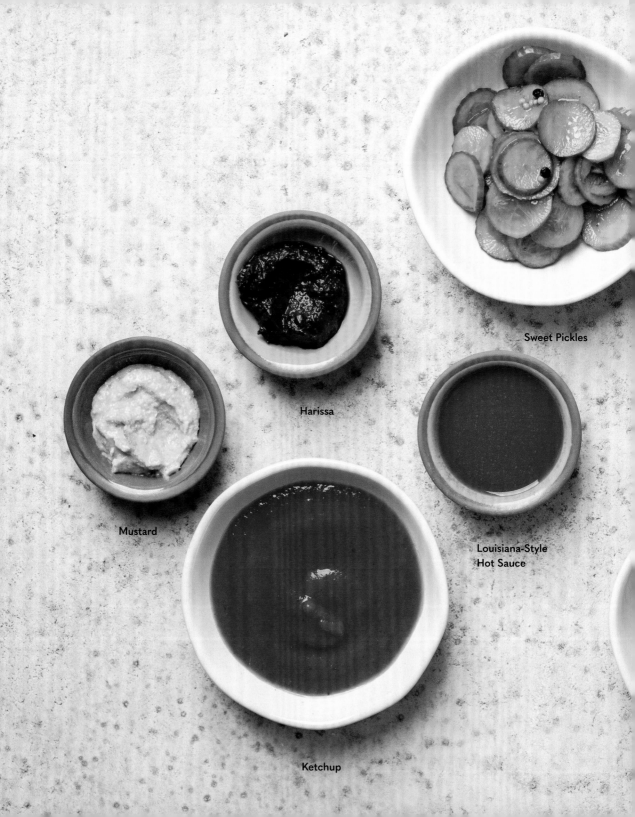

Sweet Pickles

Harissa

Mustard

Louisiana-Style
Hot Sauce

Ketchup

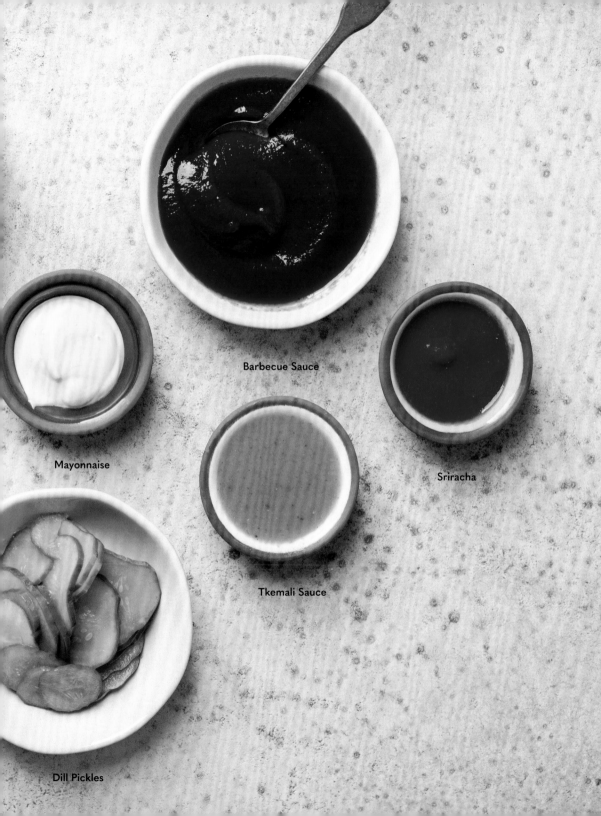

Barbecue Sauce

Mayonnaise

Sriracha

Tkemali Sauce

Dill Pickles

Tkemali Sauce

I wonder why we don't cook with plums more often. This herby-tangy-spicy Georgian sauce reminded me of just how good they are. While traditionally it's made with a type of small, green sour plum (where it gets its name), you can make this recipe with just about any plum that isn't too ripe (the riper the plums, the sweeter and less tart the sauce). This version is virtually sodium-free, so you can generously dollop it on a burger or grilled pork, or use it as a marinade, a salad dressing, or a dip for crudités.

You can play around with the dried and fresh herbs in this recipe; for example, if you don't have fresh dill, swap it out for fresh thyme. But do keep the fresh mint, as it is critical to the flavor.

Makes: About 1 cup

TOTAL SODIUM: 15 mg

SODIUM PER TABLESPOON: About 1 mg

---

1 pound firm plums (about 6)

1 cup water

3 cloves garlic, minced

2 tablespoons freshly squeezed lemon juice

2 tablespoons olive oil

1 tablespoon red wine vinegar

1 bay leaf

1 teaspoon ground coriander

1 teaspoon dried thyme

1 teaspoon fennel seed

1 teaspoon dried parsley flakes

1 teaspoon dried oregano

½ teaspoon red pepper flakes

¼ teaspoon freshly ground black pepper

2 tablespoons finely chopped fresh cilantro leaves

2 tablespoons finely chopped fresh dill

2 tablespoons finely chopped fresh mint leaves

1   With a sharp knife, score a small X on the bottom of each plum. Put them in a large saucepan over high heat with enough water to cover. Bring to a boil and blanch the plums in boiling water until the skins start to loosen, about 2 minutes. Drain them in a colander and rinse in cold water to stop the cooking. Remove the skins and the pits.

2   Return them to the saucepan with the 1 cup of water, the garlic, lemon juice, oil, vinegar, bay leaf, coriander, thyme, fennel seed, parsley, oregano, red pepper flakes, and black pepper. Simmer over medium heat until the plums are very soft, about 5 minutes. Remove the bay leaf. Add the cilantro, dill, and mint, and puree the mixture with an immersion blender or in the bowl of a food processor.

3   Return the mixture to the saucepan and simmer over medium heat until thick and flavorful, about 5 minutes. Strain through a fine-mesh sieve and allow the sauce to cool to room temperature.

4   Store in an airtight bottle or jar in the refrigerator for up to 1 month.

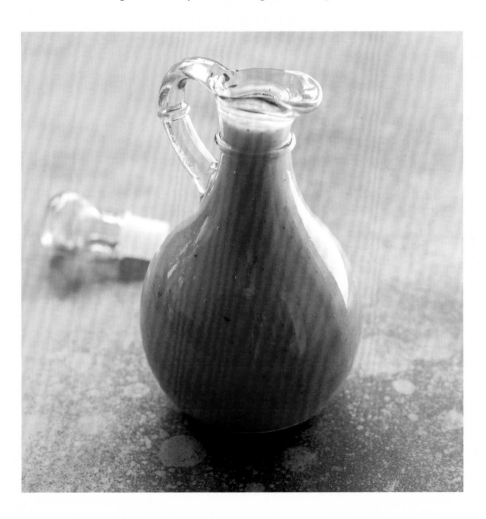

Pico de Gallo

Store-bought salsa typically comes in at around 85 milligrams per tablespoon, which, if you want to stay on target, doesn't leave much room for a little bit of salt on your chips. This fresh salsa far surpasses the packaged stuff and has only 3 milligrams per tablespoon.

A note on seeds: You can leave the seeds in the tomatoes, but your salsa will be quite wet. If you like your salsa hot, leave the seeds in the jalapeño.

Makes: About 3 cups

TOTAL SODIUM: 139 mg

SODIUM PER TABLESPOON: About 3 mg

4 plum tomatoes, seeded and chopped

1 jalapeño, seeded and minced

1 clove garlic, minced

Zest and juice of 1 medium lime

½ cup chopped red onion

½ cup coarsely chopped fresh cilantro leaves, divided

⅛ teaspoon light salt

1   In a medium bowl, combine the tomatoes, jalapeño, garlic, lime zest and juice, onion, ¼ cup of the cilantro, and the salt. Cover and let sit for 30 minutes. Stir in the remaining ¼ cup cilantro just before serving.

2   Store in an airtight container in the refrigerator for up to 3 days.

Mango Salsa

This is the recipe that lifted me out of my low-sodium depression and finally convinced me that a low-salt diet didn't mean everything had to taste blah. You really won't miss the salt in this tangy, spicy salsa. I love it as a snack, paired with sodium-free plantain chips, but it's also great on roasted pork (see page 179) and seafood (see page 191).

Makes: 2 cups
TOTAL SODIUM: 14 mg
SODIUM PER TABLESPOON:
Less than 1 mg

2 large mangoes, pitted and diced
1 jalapeño, seeded and diced (leave the seeds in for a hotter salsa)

Juice of 1 medium lime
⅓ cup diced red onion
⅓ cup chopped fresh cilantro leaves

1   In a medium bowl, combine all the ingredients. Let sit for 5 minutes before serving.

2   Store in an airtight container in the refrigerator for up to 3 days.

Sweet Pickles

These pickles have almost zero sodium! You can pile them on your burger, chop them into your tuna salad, or just serve them on a platter with crudités. Use the same brine for other vegetables that taste great in a sweet brine, such as beets, carrots, pearl onions, or turnips.

Makes: 1 pint
TOTAL SODIUM: 17 mg,
  including brine

---

1 dill frond
3 cloves garlic
3 small pickling
  cucumbers, cut into
  ¼-inch-thick slices

¾ cup apple cider
  vinegar
¼ cup water
¼ cup granulated sugar
1 teaspoon mustard
  seeds
½ teaspoon red pepper
  flakes

½ teaspoon ground
  turmeric
½ teaspoon black
  peppercorns
½ teaspoon coriander
  seeds
2 allspice berries
1 bay leaf
1 whole clove

1   Pack the dill and garlic in a pint jar, followed by the cucumbers.

2   In a small saucepan over low heat, combine the vinegar, water, sugar, mustard seeds, red pepper flakes, turmeric, peppercorns, coriander seeds, allspice berries, bay leaf, and clove. Bring to a boil, then turn off the heat.

3   Carefully ladle the hot brine into the jar, covering the cucumbers but leaving at least ½ inch of headspace. Seal the jar and let it come to room temperature. Refrigerate at least overnight before serving.

4   Store in the refrigerator for up to 2 months.

Dill Pickles

You could omit the salt in this recipe for an almost sodium-free pickle, but I think just a tiny amount really enhances the brine. Besides, each pickle has just 2 to 3 milligrams of sodium. The only way you would consume the total sodium amount listed below is if you not only ate all the pickles but also drank all the brine.

Look for small to medium Kirby or other pickling cucumbers. If you buy them from the grocery store, be sure to wash them well to remove any wax.

Makes: 1 pint

TOTAL SODIUM: 143 mg, including brine

3 dill fronds
3 cloves garlic
3 small pickling cucumbers, cut into ¼-inch-thick slices

¾ cup distilled white vinegar
¼ cup water
1 teaspoon mustard seeds
½ teaspoon granulated sugar
½ teaspoon red pepper flakes

½ teaspoon black peppercorns
½ teaspoon ground turmeric
½ teaspoon coriander seeds
⅛ teaspoon light salt
1 bay leaf

1   Pack the dill and garlic in a pint jar, followed by the cucumbers.

2   In a small saucepan over low heat, combine the vinegar, water, mustard seeds, sugar, red pepper flakes, peppercorns, turmeric, coriander seeds, salt, and bay leaf. Bring to a boil, then turn off the heat.

3   Carefully ladle the hot brine into the jar, covering the cucumbers, but leaving at least ½ inch of headspace. Seal the jar and let it come to room temperature. Refrigerate at least overnight before serving.

4   Store in the refrigerator for up to 2 months.

Salad Dressings

Classic Vinaigrette

While you could scale up this vinaigrette to keep a big batch on hand, I find it's just as easy to whip up the amount I need at the time, so this recipe makes enough for one large salad. You may notice that my vinaigrette recipes deviate from the standard oil-to-vinegar ratio. Without salt, the dressings need more acid, so increasing the vinegar helps balance the flavors.

Makes: About ¼ cup

TOTAL SODIUM: 2 mg

SODIUM PER TABLESPOON:
Less than 1 mg

2 tablespoons olive oil

2 tablespoons white or red wine vinegar

1 tablespoon freshly squeezed lemon juice

1 teaspoon minced shallot (optional)

½ teaspoon dry mustard

Freshly ground black pepper

1   Put all the ingredients in a jar with a tight-fitting lid and shake until well combined.

2   If making a larger batch, store in the refrigerator for up to 2 weeks, and shake well before each use.

Balsamic Vinaigrette

You don't need to use expensive balsamic for this vinaigrette, but do get one that has aged some, ideally at least five years, so it has the right viscosity and sweetness. Avoid imitation balsamic filled with coloring and sweeteners. I like to add some black garlic—a great source of umami to amp the flavor without the harshness of raw garlic—but you can skip it if you don't have any on hand.

Makes: About ¼ cup (enough for 1 large salad)

TOTAL SODIUM: 10 mg

SODIUM PER TABLESPOON: About 3 mg

___

2 tablespoons olive oil

2 tablespoons balsamic vinegar

1 teaspoon honey

1 teaspoon minced shallot

1 teaspoon minced black garlic (optional)

Freshly ground black pepper

1   Put all the ingredients in a jar with a tight-fitting lid and shake until well combined.

2   If making a larger batch, store in the refrigerator for up to 2 weeks, and shake well before each use.

Raspberry Vinaigrette

The '80s just called and would like their salad dressing back. Raspberry vinaigrette seems to have gone out of vogue around the same time kale salad appeared on the scene, which is too bad, because the tangy fruity dressing would be scrumptious in a kale slaw.

The beauty of this dressing is that it uses only ten raspberries, so you can snack on the rest! (Or use them in another dish, sure, if you have the willpower for that. I certainly don't.)

Makes: About ¼ cup (enough for 1 large salad)

TOTAL SODIUM: Less than 1 mg

SODIUM PER TABLESPOON: Less than 1 mg

10 raspberries

½ teaspoon granulated sugar

2 tablespoons olive oil

2 tablespoons white wine vinegar

1 tablespoon freshly squeezed lemon juice

Freshly ground black pepper

1   Put the raspberries and sugar in a small bowl and use the back of a spoon to lightly mash the berries. Let them sit for 10 minutes, then mash well.

2   Put the macerated berries, oil, vinegar, lemon juice, and pepper in a jar with a tight-fitting lid and shake until well combined.

3   If making a larger batch, store in the refrigerator for up to 2 weeks, and shake well before each use.

Green Goddess Dressing

While I was writing my book *An Avocado a Day*, I got in the habit of sneaking avocado into just about anything I could, and it really stuck for me in this creamy, herby dressing. It's a great way to use up leftover avocado, but if you leave it out, the dressing will still taste delicious.

Makes: About 1 cup

TOTAL SODIUM: 67 mg

SODIUM PER TABLESPOON: About 4 mg

1 cup fresh flat-leaf parsley leaves

¼ cup olive oil

¼ cup plain yogurt (any type)

¼ cup diced ripe avocado (optional)

3 tablespoons chopped fresh chives

2 tablespoons fresh tarragon leaves

2 tablespoons water

1 tablespoon white wine or sherry vinegar

1 clove garlic

Zest and juice of 1 medium lemon

1   Put all the ingredients in the bowl of a food processor or a blender, and blend until smooth.

2   Store in the refrigerator in an airtight container for up to 1 week, and shake well before each use.

French Dressing

I rarely eat French dressing anymore because it's got more sugar than I typically want in my salad (I'll save those calories for dessert). But it was my favorite when I was a kid, and it's a nostalgic treat to indulge in every now and then.

Makes: About 1 cup
TOTAL SODIUM: 11 mg
SODIUM PER TABLESPOON:
   Less than 1 mg

½ cup tomato puree
½ cup white wine vinegar

2 tablespoons granulated
   sugar
½ teaspoon chili powder
½ teaspoon onion
   powder

½ teaspoon dry mustard
¼ teaspoon sweet
   paprika
¼ cup olive oil

1   In a small saucepan over medium-low heat, combine the tomato puree, vinegar, sugar, chili and onion powders, mustard, and paprika, stirring until the sugar dissolves completely. Remove the pan from the heat and slowly pour in the oil, whisking thoroughly until smooth.

2   Store in the refrigerator in an airtight container for up to 2 weeks, and shake well before each use.

Lemon Cream Dressing

To me, the perfect salad is made from Little Gem lettuce (a hybrid that is like a combination of butter and romaine lettuces) with a generous portion of lemon cream dressing. This recipe, which I adapted from the wonderful one in Joshua McFadden's cookbook, *Six Seasons: A New Way with Vegetables*, is terrific even without any salt.

Makes: About ½ cup

TOTAL SODIUM: 45 mg

SODIUM PER TABLESPOON: About 6 mg

4 cloves garlic, smashed
½ cup heavy cream
½ teaspoon freshly ground black pepper

3 tablespoons olive oil
2 tablespoons freshly squeezed lemon juice

1   In a small bowl, combine the garlic, cream, and pepper. Cover and chill for 1 hour.

2   After 1 hour, strain the cream mixture through a fine-mesh sieve into a jar with a tight-fitting lid, discarding the garlic or reserving it for another use. Add the oil and shake until thickened, then add the lemon juice and shake to combine.

3   Store in the refrigerator in an airtight container for up to 4 days, and shake well before each use.

Ranch Dressing

Ranch dressing's iconic tang comes from buttermilk. If you don't have buttermilk, you can substitute the same quantity of regular milk with a teaspoon of lemon juice mixed in. Your dressing will be a little thinner, but still tasty. Of course, this is great on salad, but also try it as a dipping sauce for the Crispy Sweet Potato Wedges (page 214).

Makes: About 1 cup
TOTAL SODIUM: 135 mg
SODIUM PER TABLESPOON:
About 8 mg

½ cup Greek yogurt
⅓ cup buttermilk
1 tablespoon olive oil

1 teaspoon dried chives, or 1 tablespoon chopped fresh
1 teaspoon dried parsley flakes, or 1 tablespoon chopped fresh flat-leaf parsley leaves
1 teaspoon freshly squeezed lemon juice

½ teaspoon dried or fresh dill
¼ teaspoon sweet paprika
1 clove garlic, minced
Freshly ground black pepper

1   Put all the ingredients in the bowl of a food processor or a blender, and blend until smooth.

2   Store in the refrigerator in an airtight container for up to 1 week, and shake well before each use.

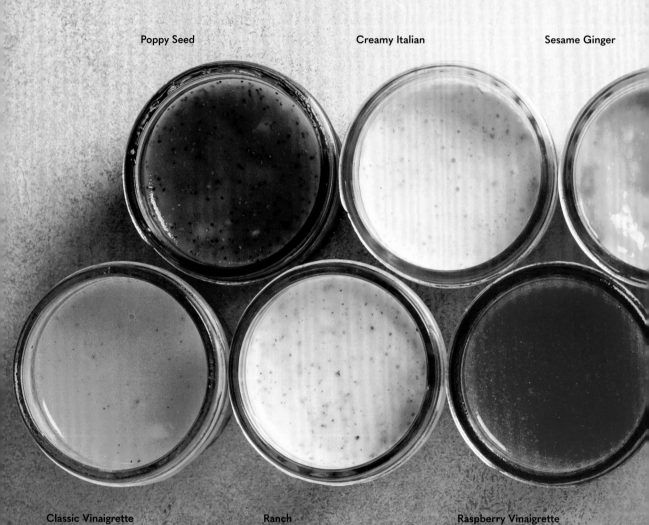

Poppy Seed

Creamy Italian

Sesame Ginger

Classic Vinaigrette

Ranch

Raspberry Vinaigrette

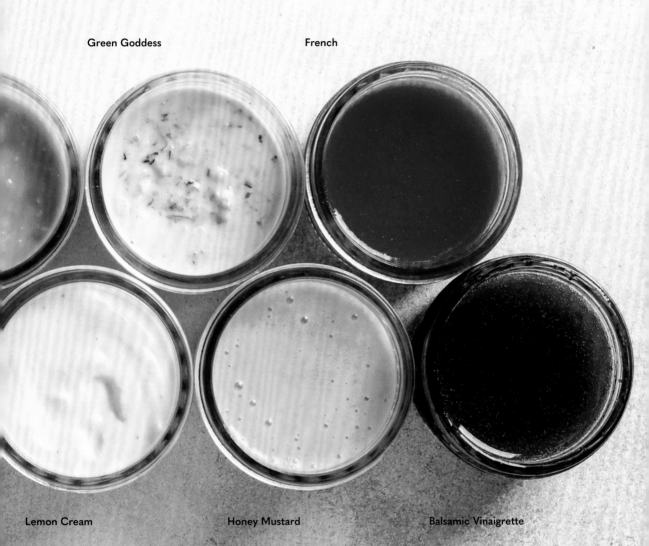

Green Goddess

French

Lemon Cream

Honey Mustard

Balsamic Vinaigrette

Poppy Seed Dressing

Try this dressing with shredded cabbage and matchstick apple pieces for a great low-sodium coleslaw, which pairs well with Barbecue Ribs (page 182).

Makes: About ½ cup

TOTAL SODIUM: 25 mg

SODIUM PER TABLESPOON:
   About 3 mg

_____

½ cup olive oil

¼ cup red wine vinegar

2 tablespoons honey or granulated sugar

1 tablespoon Mustard (page 4)

1 tablespoon poppy seeds

1 teaspoon minced shallot

1   Put all the ingredients in a jar with a tight-fitting lid and shake until well combined.

2   Store in the refrigerator in an airtight container for up to 2 weeks, and shake well before each use.

Honey Mustard Dressing

Although you can use any low-sodium mustard for this dressing, I prefer a lighter (more yellow) mustard for salads—especially spinach. If you are making this for a sandwich spread, using a whole grain brown mustard is really nice.

Makes: About ½ cup

TOTAL SODIUM: 35 mg

SODIUM PER TABLESPOON:
  About 4 mg

3 tablespoons honey

3 tablespoons apple
  cider vinegar

2 tablespoons olive oil

2 tablespoons Mustard
  (page 4)

1   Put all the ingredients in a food processor or blender, and blend until smooth.

2   Store in the refrigerator in an airtight container for up to 2 weeks, and shake well before each use.

Creamy Italian Dressing

This is a great dressing for simple butter-lettuce salads, as well as chopped salads with multiple ingredients, such as Vegetable Chopped Salad (page 134). It keeps well in the refrigerator and is a little lighter than ranch dressing.

Makes: About ½ cup

TOTAL SODIUM: 47 mg

SODIUM PER TABLESPOON: About 6 mg

¼ cup plain yogurt (any type)

2 tablespoons olive oil

2 tablespoons white wine vinegar

1 teaspoon minced shallot

1 teaspoon Mustard (page 4)

1 teaspoon dried parsley flakes, or 1 tablespoon chopped fresh flat-leaf parsley leaves

1 teaspoon dried or fresh basil

½ teaspoon minced garlic

Pinch of red pepper flakes

1   Put all the ingredients in a food processor or blender, and blend until smooth.

2   Store in the refrigerator in an airtight container for up to 2 weeks, and shake well before each use.

Sesame Ginger Dressing

In college, I lived on Annie's Sesame Ginger Vinaigrette (along with other high-sodium college staples, such as ramen and mac and cheese). Annie's version has 125 milligrams of sodium per tablespoon, but this recipe only has 12 milligrams.

Be sure to check your rice vinegar and tahini labels to make sure they aren't seasoned with extra sugar and salt.

Makes: About ½ cup
TOTAL SODIUM: 92 mg
SODIUM PER TABLESPOON:
About 12 mg

___

3 tablespoons toasted sesame oil
3 tablespoons olive oil

3 tablespoons unseasoned rice vinegar
1½ tablespoons lightly packed light brown sugar

1½ tablespoons tahini
1 tablespoon minced ginger
1 teaspoon coconut aminos
1 clove garlic, minced

1   Put all the ingredients in a food processor or blender, and blend until smooth.

2   Store in the refrigerator in an airtight container for up to 2 weeks, and shake well before each use.

Spice Blends

Popcorn Seasoning

After a few bowls of popcorn with this seasoning, you may wonder why you ever thought salt was enough of a flavoring. This spice mixture is a little tangy, a little smoky, and a little buttery—and, I think, a whole lot more worthy of finger-licking.

Makes: Enough for 2 large bowls of popcorn (about 10 cups)

TOTAL SODIUM: 3 mg

2 tablespoons sumac

2 tablespoons *amchoor* powder

1 teaspoon smoked paprika

1 teaspoon ground peppercorns

1   In a small bowl, combine all the ingredients. Generously sprinkle on your buttered (or not) popcorn.

2   Store in an airtight container at room temperature for up to 6 months.

Barbecue Dry Rub

If you're like me, you tend to forget to plan time for marinating. Enter the dry rub. Just rub it into the meat and then grill, broil, or roast—no need to plan ahead. Take this recipe as a framework: it has the smoky, sweet, and spicy basics, but you can add in other flavors or increase the heat (this rub is on the mild side).

Makes: About 1 cup

TOTAL SODIUM: 536 mg

SODIUM PER TABLESPOON: About 34 mg

¼ cup smoked paprika

¼ cup lightly packed light brown sugar

¼ cup salt-free chili powder

2 tablespoons coriander seeds

1 tablespoon cumin seeds

1 tablespoon fennel seeds

1 tablespoon red pepper flakes

1 teaspoon freshly ground black pepper

1 teaspoon dried rosemary

½ teaspoon light salt

1   In a food processor, combine all the ingredients and pulse until finely ground.

2   Store in an airtight container at room temperature for up to 6 months.

Taco Seasoning

Taco-seasoning packets are full of salt: just two teaspoons of one of the leading brands has 380 milligrams of sodium. This seasoning has very little sodium, but your tacos will still be happy! Use it like you would those packets: mixed with ground beef, simmered into chicken tortilla soup, or combined with sour cream for a dip. Substitute two tablespoons for one seasoning packet.

Makes: About 1 cup
TOTAL SODIUM: 83 mg
SODIUM PER TABLESPOON:
About 5 mg

———

3 dried guajillo chilies, stemmed, seeded, and chopped

3 dried ancho chilies, stemmed, seeded, and chopped

3 dried arbol chilies, stemmed, seeded, and chopped

2 tablespoons cumin seeds

2 tablespoons garlic powder

1 tablespoon onion powder

1 tablespoon dried oregano

1 teaspoon smoked paprika

1 teaspoon cornstarch

1   In a food processor, combine all the ingredients and pulse until finely ground.

2   Store in an airtight container at room temperature for up to 6 months.

Lemon Pepper

Lemon pepper is a go-to spice mix for those reducing salt, but store-bought versions can get stale and sometimes tastes more like dried grass than seasoning. Just as freshly ground black pepper is far more flavorful than preground, blending your own lemon pepper from scratch is a revelation.

If you don't want to dry your own zest, you can order ground lemon zest online.

Makes: About ⅓ cup

TOTAL SODIUM: Less than 1 mg

SODIUM PER TABLESPOON: 0 mg

Zest of 3 medium lemons (about 3 tablespoons)
1 tablespoon white or black peppercorns
1 teaspoon dried oregano
½ teaspoon citric acid
½ teaspoon red pepper flakes
¼ teaspoon sumac

1   Line a baking sheet with parchment paper, spread the zest out on the sheet, and heat in the oven at its lowest setting until the zest is dried, 25 to 35 minutes.

2   In a spice grinder, combine the dried zest with the remaining ingredients and pulse until finely ground.

3   Store in an airtight container at room temperature for up to 6 months.

Cajun Seasoning

You should definitely use this seasoning for blackened pan-fried fish fillets, but it's also great on potatoes (try adding it to the Hash Browns on page 129) or mixed into rice. This mix is pretty spicy, so if you need to dial back the heat, cut down on the amount of cayenne pepper.

Makes: About ½ cup
TOTAL SODIUM: 39 mg
SODIUM PER TABLESPOON:
About 5 mg

1 ancho chili, stemmed, seeded, and chopped
2 tablespoons cayenne pepper
2 tablespoons garlic powder
2 tablespoons sweet paprika
1 tablespoon dried oregano
1 tablespoon dried thyme
1 tablespoon freshly ground black pepper
1 tablespoon onion powder
Pinch of ground bay leaf

1   In a food processor, combine all the ingredients and pulse until finely ground.

2   Store in an airtight container at room temperature for up to 6 months.

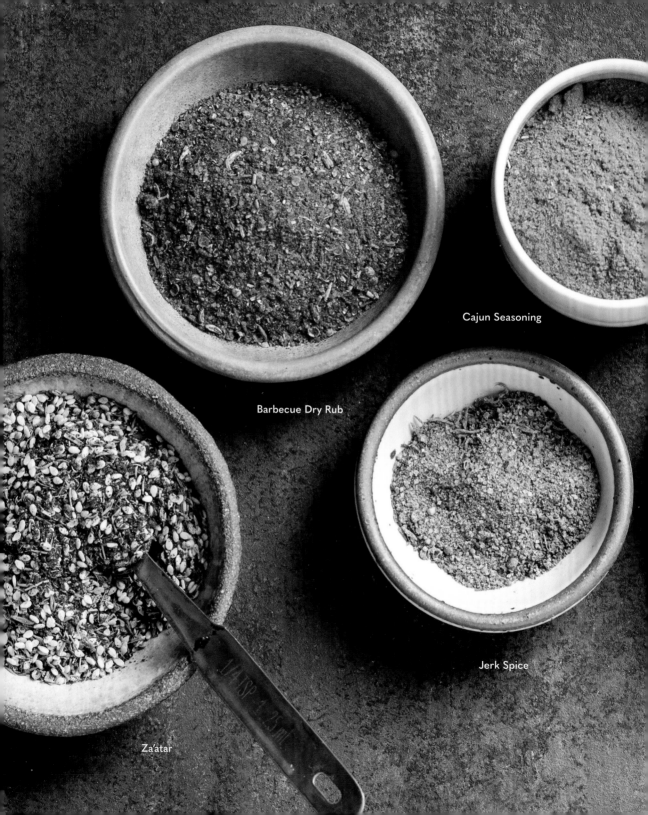

Cajun Seasoning

Barbecue Dry Rub

Jerk Spice

Za'atar

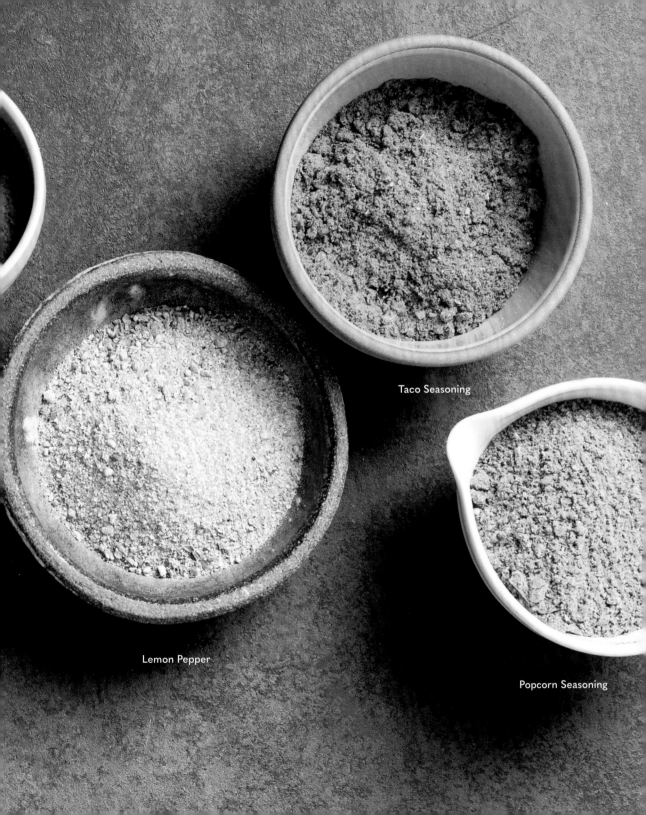

Taco Seasoning

Lemon Pepper

Popcorn Seasoning

Jerk Spice

This almost zero-sodium spice mix packs a lot of flavor. It's great on grilled fish, chicken, pork, or even grilled vegetables, especially cauliflower, green beans, or sweet potatoes. Just brush a bit of olive oil on whatever you're grilling before sprinkling it on.

If you're cutting back on sugar, you can swap it out for a substitute such as monk fruit granules, or even leave it out, but you won't get the same browning effect.

Makes: About ½ cup
TOTAL SODIUM: 11 mg
SODIUM PER TABLESPOON:
About 1 mg

2 tablespoons granulated sugar

1 tablespoon plus 1 teaspoon dried thyme

2 teaspoons ground allspice

2 teaspoons freshly ground black pepper

2 teaspoons onion powder

2 teaspoons sweet paprika

2 teaspoons dried parsley flakes

2 teaspoons ground ginger

1 teaspoon cayenne pepper

1 teaspoon garlic powder

½ teaspoon freshly grated nutmeg

½ teaspoon ground cinnamon

1   In a food processor, combine all the ingredients and pulse until finely ground.

2   Store in an airtight container at room temperature for up to 6 months.

Za'atar

You could omit or reduce the salt in this Middle Eastern spice mix, which is mostly sumac, thyme, and sesame, but I think the salt here really helps boost the flavor while still keeping the recipe reasonably low sodium. Consider making a double batch so you have it around to garnish hummus, yogurt, potatoes, or eggs.

Makes: About ½ cup
TOTAL SODIUM: 255 mg
SODIUM PER TABLESPOON:
   About 32 mg
⅄⁄⁄
¼ cup sumac

¼ cup toasted sesame
   seeds
2 tablespoons dried
   thyme

1 tablespoon dried
   oregano
¼ teaspoon light salt

1   Mix all the ingredients in a mortar and lightly crush them with a pestle to release the oils in the sesame seeds. Alternatively, you can quickly pulse them a few times in a food processor.

2   Store in an airtight container at room temperature for up to 6 months.

Baked Goods

Honey Whole Wheat Sandwich Bread

This is my favorite sandwich bread. It's beautifully soft when freshly baked and toasts up well for grilled or toasted sandwiches. The honey and whole wheat add just the right amount of flavor, which can be missing in low-sodium breads. It's also amazing simply slathered in jam.

Makes: 2 loaves
SODIUM PER LOAF: 177 mg
SODIUM PER SLICE: About 15 mg

1 tablespoon vegetable oil, for greasing
3 cups warm water (80 degrees F)

2 tablespoons honey
2 tablespoons dry milk powder
4 teaspoons (2 packets) active dry yeast
5¾ cups (700 grams) all-purpose flour

2½ cups (300 grams) whole wheat flour
¼ teaspoon light salt
2 teaspoons unsalted butter, melted (optional)

DO AHEAD: If you won't go through 2 loaves in a few days, parbake the bread: bake until the loaves are pale golden, about 20 minutes. Let the loaves cool completely (at least 2 hours), then wrap them tightly in plastic wrap and freeze. When you're ready to use them, unwrap the loaves and bake, still frozen, in a 450-degree-F oven for 20 minutes.

1   Lightly grease a large bowl (at least twice the size of the dough) and two 8½-by-4½-by-3-inch loaf pans with the oil.

2   Put the warm water, honey, and milk powder in the bowl of a stand mixer. Sprinkle the yeast on top and stir to dissolve.

3   Add the all-purpose and whole wheat flours, and the salt. Using the dough hook attachment, knead on the lowest speed until most of the flour is wet and the mixture starts to form a dough, about 1 minute. Increase the speed to medium and knead for 1 more minute. Increase the speed to high and knead for another 4 minutes. The dough should be smooth and the sides of the bowl clean.

continued

4   Turn the dough out onto a lightly floured work surface. Using clean hands, gently flatten the dough and fold it 3 to 4 times. Shape it into a ball, and place the ball in the prepared bowl. Lightly grease the top of the dough. Cover it with a damp towel and let it sit in a warm spot (75 to 80 degrees F) for 40 minutes, until doubled in size. Punch down the dough, then cover it again and let it continue to rise until doubled in size, another 40 minutes.

5   Turn the dough out onto a lightly floured work surface, and using a sharp knife or bench scraper, divide the dough into two equally weighted pieces. Gently shape each piece into a round loaf, dust each loaf lightly with flour, and cover.

6   Gently flatten one of the loaves on a lightly floured surface to form an 8-by-12-inch rectangle. Place the narrow side closest to you and roll from the bottom edge to form a log. Pinch the seam to seal. Then pull each end of the log down and underneath to form a smooth loaf. Pinch to seal, and place in the greased pan with the seam down. Repeat with the other dough ball.

7   Cover each loaf loosely with plastic wrap and let it rest in a warm spot until the dough has risen to just above the edge of the pan, about 40 minutes.

8   While the dough is rising, preheat the oven to 400 degrees F with the rack in the middle position.

9   After the dough has risen, gently brush the top of each loaf with the melted butter (or, alternatively, dust with a bit of flour). Bake until the top of the bread is a deep golden brown, about 40 minutes.

Variation: Hamburger Buns

This dough also makes terrific burger buns. Make the dough as directed, but instead of forming it into two loaves, divide the dough into 24 equal pieces. Form each piece into a 3-inch round, and lightly flatten. Put the buns on a parchment paper–lined baking sheet, leaving ½ inch between them. Cover with a damp towel and let rise in a warm spot for 1 hour. Preheat the oven to 375 degrees F. Brush the top of each bun with some melted butter, and bake until deep golden brown, 12 to 18 minutes. Cool on a wire rack.

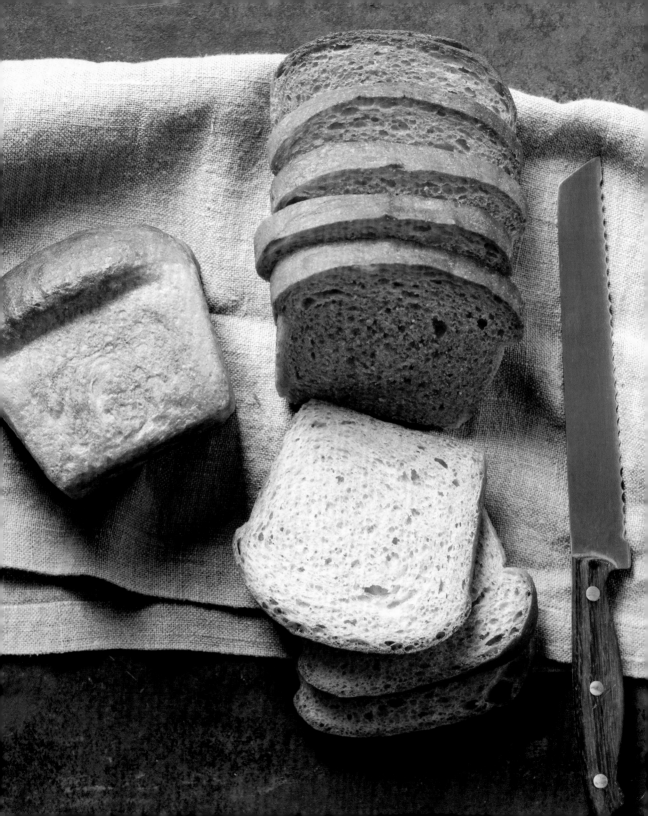

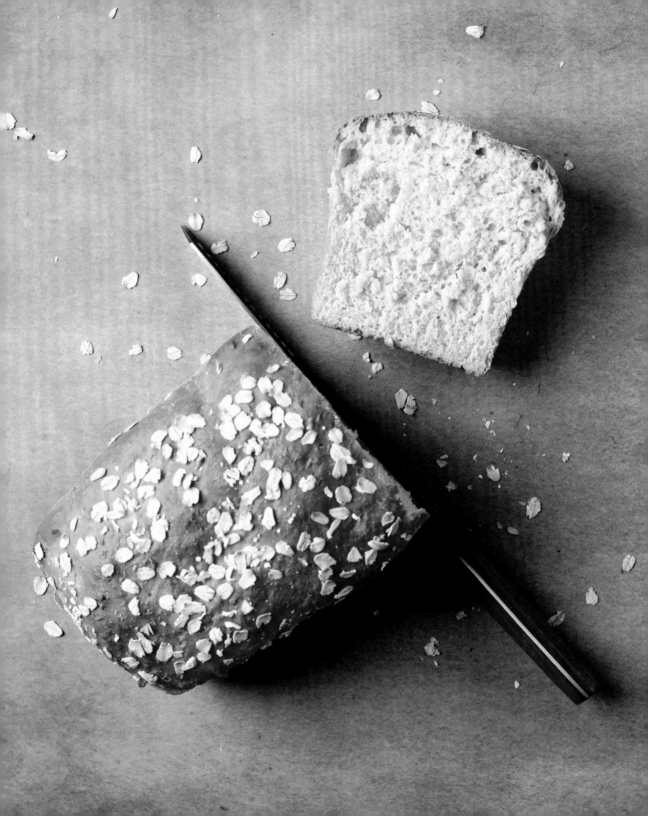

Oatmeal Batter Bread

If you are new to baking with yeast, don't have a lot of time for baking, or just want a really delicious slice of toast for your breakfast, this is a great bread recipe to start with. Unlike most yeast breads, this loaf requires no kneading or shaping, and the rising time is relatively short. It also makes great French toast!

Makes: 1 loaf

TOTAL SODIUM: 345 mg

SODIUM PER SLICE: About 29 mg

1 teaspoon vegetable oil or unsalted butter, for greasing

2½ cups (300 grams) all-purpose flour, divided

¾ cup plus 1 tablespoon rolled oats, divided

2 heaping teaspoons (1 packet) active dry yeast

¼ teaspoon light salt

1 cup warm water (80 degrees F)

2 tablespoons honey

¼ cup unsalted butter

1 tablespoon apple cider vinegar

1 large egg

1   Lightly grease an 8½-by-4½-by-3-inch loaf pan with the oil.

2   In the bowl of a stand mixer, gently whisk together the flour, ¾ cup of the oats, the yeast, and salt. Set aside.

3   In a small saucepan, warm the water, honey, and butter over medium-low heat, stirring occasionally, just until the butter melts. You can also do this in the microwave.

4   Add the warmed butter mixture to the flour, along with the vinegar and egg. Using the paddle attachment, mix on low speed until the flour is moistened, about 1 minute. Beat on medium-high for 3 minutes. The batter will be stiff, but still pretty sticky. Cover the bowl with a damp towel and let the dough rise for 30 to 45 minutes, until doubled in size.

5   Preheat the oven to 375 degrees F.

continued

6   Spoon the batter into the loaf pan, and sprinkle the remaining 1 tablespoon of oats on top. Loosely cover the loaf with plastic wrap and let it rise for 15 to 25 minutes, or until the dough has risen just above the edge of the pan.

7   Bake the bread until it is golden brown, about 30 minutes. Turn it out onto a wire rack and allow it to cool for at least 20 minutes before slicing.

8   Store the cooled bread in a plastic bag (it will soften) at room temperature for up to 3 days.

9   To freeze the bread, allow it to cool completely, then slice it and wrap it tightly in plastic wrap. To use, toast from frozen or defrost in the refrigerator.

Baguette

I got my love of baking bread from my dad, who taught me how to properly knead dough, and I make these simple baguettes more than any other loaf. These days, I tend to leave the kneading up to my stand mixer, but I still get my hands in on the action by shaping the baguettes. Getting the right surface tension and slashes in the dough can take a while to master, so don't fret if your loaf cracks a little. You'll be enjoying it so much you won't notice.

A bit of rye flour in the mix adds some hearty, country-loaf flavor to this recipe, but if you don't have any, feel free to use all bread flour, or the same amount of whole wheat flour.

Makes: 2 baguettes

SODIUM PER BAGUETTE:
259 mg

SODIUM PER SLICE: About
13 mg

10 ounces warm water (90 degrees F)

1 teaspoon apple cider vinegar

2 teaspoons (1 packet) active dry yeast

3⅓ cups (400 grams) bread flour

½ cup (50 grams) rye flour or bread flour

½ teaspoon light salt

DO AHEAD: If you won't go through 2 baguettes in a few days, parbake the bread: bake for only 8 minutes after venting the steam instead of 10 to 15. The loaves should be a pale golden color. Let the loaves cool completely (at least 2 hours), then wrap them tightly in plastic wrap and freeze. When you're ready to use them, unwrap the loaves and bake, still frozen, in a 450-degree-F oven for 20 minutes.

1   Pour the warm water and vinegar into the bowl of a stand mixer. Sprinkle the yeast on top and stir to dissolve. Add the bread and rye flours, and the salt.

2   Using the dough hook attachment, knead on the lowest speed until most of the flour is wet and the mixture starts to form a dough, about 1 minute. Increase the speed to medium and knead for 1 more minute. Increase the speed to high and knead for another 4 minutes.

continued

3   Turn the dough out onto a lightly floured work surface. Using clean hands, gently flatten the dough and fold it a few times. Return the dough to the mixer, and knead it on medium speed for another 2 minutes until smooth.

4   Turn the dough out again onto the work surface, adding more flour if needed. Using clean hands, gently flatten the dough and fold it 3 or 4 times. Form it into a ball, and place the ball in a large bowl. Cover it with plastic wrap and let it sit in a warm spot (75 to 80 degrees F) for at least 1 hour until the dough has doubled. Let it rest for up to 3 hours, if possible, to develop more flavor.

5   Line a baking sheet with parchment paper.

6   Turn the dough out again onto the work surface, adding more flour if needed. Using a sharp knife or bench scraper, divide the dough into two equally weighted pieces. Gently shape one of the loaves into a 6-by-10-inch rectangle, with the short side facing you. Fold the top of the dough down to the center, and the bottom of the dough up to the center. Then take the new top of the dough and fold it down to the bottom edge of the dough. Pinch to seal. Place the dough, seam side down, on the baking sheet. Repeat with the remaining loaf. Loosely cover the loaves with plastic wrap and let them rest for 40 minutes, until the dough has risen by 50 percent.

7   When the dough has rested, uncover one of the loaves and place it on a flour-free surface, with the long side facing you. Pull the top of the dough to meet the bottom edge, and pinch along the edge to seal. Rotate the loaf until it is seam side up. Push down on the seam with the side of your hand to create a crease. Then pull the top edge over the crease, down to meet the bottom edge. Pinch to seal. You should have a long cylinder. Gently roll the cylinder until it is about 12 inches long. Return the cylinder to the baking sheet. Repeat with the other loaf. Sprinkle the loaves with a little flour. Cover them loosely with plastic wrap (the flour will keep the plastic wrap from sticking to them), and let them rest for 30 to 45 minutes until the dough has risen by about 25 percent.

8   While the dough is resting, preheat the oven to 500 degrees F. Place a rack in the middle position and another rack below it. Place an oven-safe skillet on the lower rack.

9   Remove the plastic wrap from the loaves and let them sit uncovered for 5 minutes so the surface dries slightly. Then, using a bread *lame* or serrated knife, make 4 or 5 (¼-inch-deep) diagonal slashes along the top of each cylinder.

continued

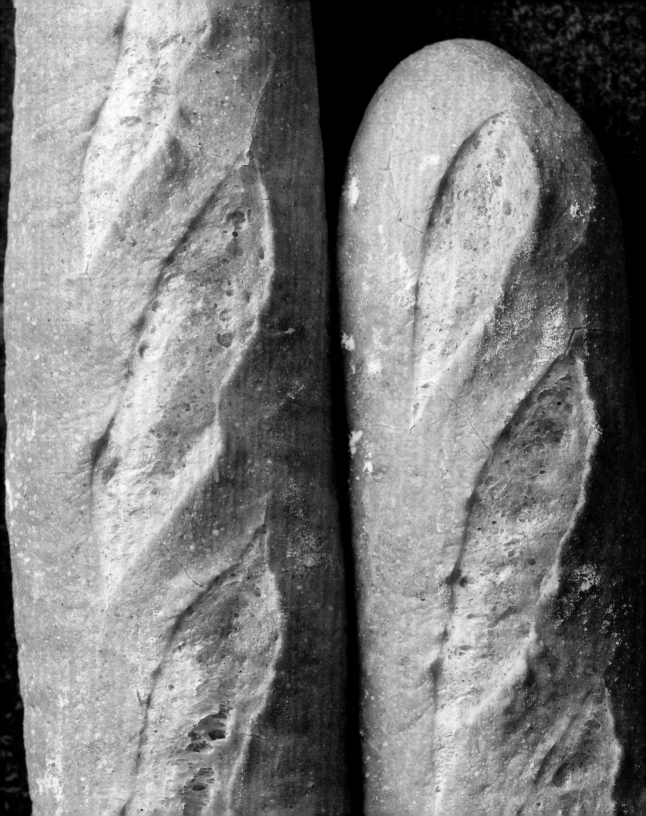

10 Reduce the oven temperature to 450 degrees F. Transfer the baking sheet to the top rack of the oven and pour about ½ cup of water into the skillet. (This will create steam and help improve the quality of the crust.) Close the oven door and bake for 10 minutes. Then open the oven door for 1 minute to vent the steam. Close the door again, and continue to bake until the crust is a deep golden brown, 10 to 15 minutes.

11 Transfer the loaves to a wire rack and allow to cool completely before cutting.

12 The baguettes are best eaten on the day they are baked. To store them, wrap them in plastic wrap and store at room temperature. The crust will get soft, so re-crisp it by heating the bread in a 350-degree oven for about 5 minutes before serving.

Variation: Bread Crumbs

You can make bread crumbs from the Honey Whole Wheat Sandwich Bread (page 43), but I especially like using these baguettes.

Leave the bread out, unwrapped, on the counter overnight or toast it in a 200-degree oven until hard, about 20 minutes. Chop it into chunks, then pulse the chunks in a food processor to create crumbs. If your bread wasn't completely dry, spread the bread crumbs on a parchment paper–lined baking sheet, and toast in a 200-degree oven until they are dry to help them keep longer. Store in an airtight container at room temperature for 1 month, or freeze for up to 2 months.

Bagels

These bagels stay fresh longer, thanks to insights I gleaned from Stella Parks's bagel recipe on Serious Eats. She was inspired by a Japanese roux called *yudane*, which precooks a small amount of the flour before making the dough. This step helps the dough retain moisture so the bagels don't go stale as easily. However, her recipe uses a lot of salt: about 350 milligrams per bagel. Because of the long fermentation, most of the salt can be cut without sacrificing flavor—there's only 27 milligrams per bagel without any toppings, so you don't have to worry about spreading on some Cream Cheese (page 109). Toppings such as sesame seeds, poppy seeds, and *shichimi togarashi* are low in sodium, or try the Za'atar (page 41).

Barley malt syrup gives bagels their distinctive, subtle nutty sweetness, but you can substitute honey or molasses. The bagels need to rest for at least twenty-four hours in the refrigerator to develop flavor before cooking, so make sure you have room for a baking sheet, and plan your time accordingly.

Makes: 10 bagels

TOTAL SODIUM: 268 mg

SODIUM PER BAGEL:
  About 27 mg (without toppings)

1½ cups water, divided

3¾ cups (450 grams) bread flour, divided

1 tablespoon granulated sugar

1 teaspoon active dry yeast

¼ teaspoon light salt

1 tablespoon barley malt syrup or honey

1   First, make the *yudane*: In a small saucepan over medium heat, stir 1 cup of the water with 1 cup (120 grams) of the flour until combined. Continue to cook until the mixture thickens to a stiff paste, 1 to 2 minutes. Transfer the *yudane* to the bowl of a stand mixer and let it cool for 30 to 40 minutes to about 80 degrees F, or barely warm to the touch.

2   When the *yudane* is almost cooled, in a small bowl, mix the remaining ½ cup of water with the sugar and yeast. Let it sit for about 5 minutes to activate the yeast.

continued

3   Add the yeast mixture to the cooled *yudane*, then add the remaining 2¾ cups flour (330 grams) and salt. Using the dough hook attachment, knead on low speed for 2 minutes. Increase the speed to medium and knead until you have a smooth, very stiff dough, another 2 minutes.

4   Turn the dough out onto a lightly floured work surface. Using a sharp knife or bench scraper, divide the dough into 10 equal pieces (about 70 grams each). Working with one piece at a time, put the dough on a flour-free work surface. Place your hand over the dough with your fingertips just touching the work surface and your palm resting on the dough. Move your hand in a circle to roll the dough into a smooth ball with just a small seam on the bottom. Pinch the seam to seal. Repeat with the remaining dough pieces. Cover loosely with plastic wrap and let rest for 15 minutes.

5   Line a baking sheet with parchment paper and set it aside. Make sure there is enough room in your refrigerator to accommodate the baking sheet.

6   With a lightly damp finger, poke a hole in the center of each dough ball. Gently stretch the dough so the hole is about 2 inches wide. Put the bagels on the baking sheet, leaving at least 1 inch between them. Cover the sheet with plastic wrap and refrigerate for at least 24 hours and up to 36 hours.

7   When you are ready to bake the bagels, preheat the oven to 400 degrees F.

8   Fill a medium pot (at least 3-quart capacity), with about 3 inches of water and bring the water to a boil over high heat. Line a baking sheet with a non-terry towel, and line another baking sheet with parchment paper (you can reuse the parchment the bagels were refrigerated on).

9   When the water boils, stir in the barley malt syrup or honey. Using a spatula, carefully place two bagels in the water, and boil for about 30 seconds on each side. Transfer the bagels to the towel and let sit to remove some of the water, then transfer to the parchment-lined baking sheet. Repeat with the remaining bagels.

10 If you'd like to add toppings on your bagel, add them now, rewetting the top of the bagel if needed to get the toppings to stick. Bake until deep golden brown, about 20 minutes. Allow to cool on a wire rack for at least 15 minutes before serving.

11 Store uncut bagels at room temperature in a paper bag for up to 2 days.

12 To freeze the bagels, allow them to cool completely, then wrap them tightly in plastic wrap. To reheat, toast from frozen in a 350-degree oven for 15 minutes.

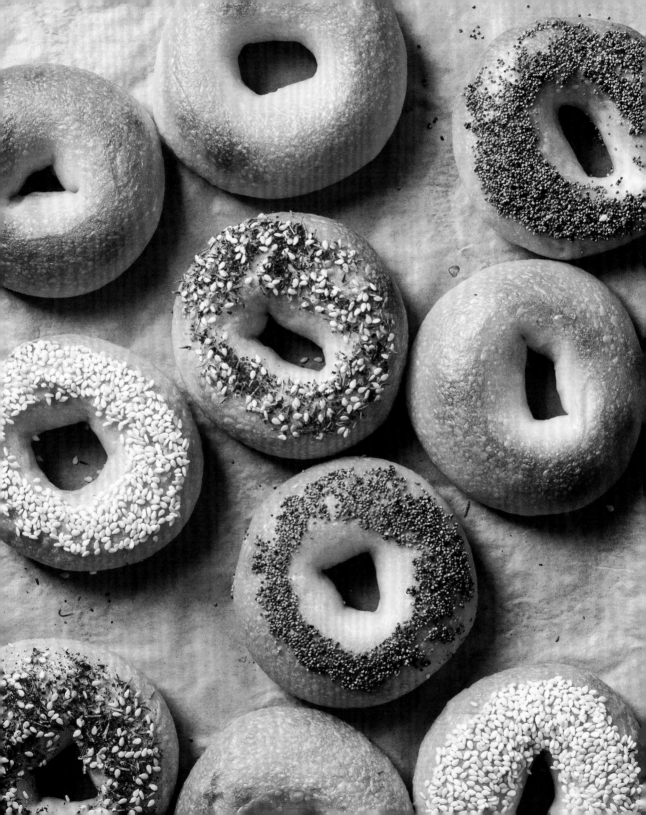

Focaccia

Whether plain, made savory topped with herbs or vegetables, or made sweet topped with grapes or cherries, this bread is a delicious accompaniment to most meals. It even makes for a great light lunch on its own. Great low-sodium topping options include chopped rosemary, red pepper flakes, sliced onion, cherry tomato halves, or mushrooms.

Makes: 2 focaccias

SODIUM PER FOCACCIA:
138 mg

SODIUM PER SLICE: About
15 mg

2 cups warm water (105 degrees F)
1 tablespoon active dry yeast
1½ tablespoons granulated sugar or honey

5¼ cups (630 grams) bread flour, plus more for dusting
¾ cup plus 2 tablespoons olive oil, plus more for greasing, divided
¼ teaspoon light salt

DO AHEAD: If you won't go through both focaccias in a few days, parbake one: bake only until pale golden, about 10 minutes. Let the focaccia cool completely (at least 2 hours), then wrap it tightly in plastic wrap and freeze. When you're ready to serve it, unwrap and bake the focaccia, still frozen, in a 450-degree-F oven for 15 minutes.

1   Pour the water into the bowl of a stand mixer and sprinkle the yeast on top. Stir in the sugar. Add the flour, ½ cup of the olive oil, and the salt.

2   Using the dough hook attachment, knead on the lowest speed until most of the flour is wet and the mixture starts to form a dough, about 1 minute. Increase the speed to medium and knead for 1 more minute. Increase the speed to high and knead for another 4 minutes.

3   Turn the dough out onto a lightly floured work surface. Using clean hands, gently flatten the dough and fold it a few times. Return it to the mixer, and knead another 2 minutes on medium speed.

4   Return the dough to the work surface. Using clean hands, gently flatten the dough and fold it a few times. Form it into a ball, and place the ball in a large bowl. Cover it with plastic wrap and let it sit in a warm spot (75 to 80 degrees F) for 1 hour, until doubled.

5   Turn the dough out again onto the work surface, adding more flour if needed. Using a sharp knife or bench scraper, divide the dough into two equally weighted pieces. Using clean hands, shape each piece into a ball, and lightly oil the top of each. Cover with plastic wrap and let rest on the work surface for another 30 minutes. The dough may rise slightly.

6   Preheat the oven to 450 degrees F. Grease two 9-by-13-inch baking sheets with ¼ cup of the oil, splitting it equally between them.

7   Place a dough ball on each of the oiled baking sheets and, using your fingertips, spread the dough to fit the sheet and poke indentations across the surface as you go. Makes sure that the whole surface is dimpled. If you'd like to add toppings, scatter them evenly over the dough.

8   Cover with plastic wrap and let rise in a warm place (75 to 80 degrees F) for 30 minutes.

9   Drizzle 1 tablespoon of the remaining olive oil over each focaccia sheet. Bake until golden brown on top and bottom, 14 to 15 minutes. Serve warm.

10 Focaccia is best eaten on the day it's made. To store focaccia, wrap each sheet in plastic wrap and keep at room temperature for up to 2 days. The crust will get soft, so re-crisp it by heating in a 350-degree oven for about 5 minutes before serving.

Pizza Dough

Pizza is probably the one food I missed more than any other after going low sodium. Just a slice or two would put me way over my daily limit. Between the sodium in the dough and sauce, not to mention all the cheese or salty meats, I might as well just have eaten a spoonful of salt.

Luckily, you can make a terrific pizza without much sodium, and it starts with this pizza dough. To develop the most flavor, I let the dough ferment slowly—at least eight hours. It's tempting to take a short cut and skip this step, but since there's little salt in this recipe, without fermentation, you may be disappointed in the flavor. So plan ahead and start the dough at least the night before you want to make pizza.

As well, the dough needs to come to room temperature before you bake the pizza, so take it out of the refrigerator two hours before you plan to put it in the oven.

Makes: Enough dough for four 12-inch pizzas

SODIUM PER PIZZA
DOUGH: 129 mg

3½ cups (420 grams) all-purpose flour, plus more for dusting

1 tablespoon granulated sugar
1 teaspoon active dry yeast
½ teaspoon light salt

1½ cups warm water (80 degrees F)
¼ cup olive oil
1 tablespoon apple cider vinegar

1   In the bowl of a stand mixer fitted with the dough hook attachment, combine the flour, sugar, yeast, and salt. In a small bowl, mix the water, oil, and vinegar.

2   With the mixer on low speed, pour in the water mixture, and knead until a dough forms, about 2 minutes. Increase the speed to high and knead, adding a bit more flour if needed, until the dough forms a ball and pulls away from the sides of the bowl, about 5 minutes.

3   Dust a large lidded bowl with a generous sprinkling of flour. Place the dough in the bowl and, using clean hands, fold it a few times. Dust the top with more flour, cover the bowl, and refrigerate for at least 8 hours and up to 3 days.

4   Before you are ready to bake, remove the dough from the refrigerator and let sit in a warm place (70 to 80 degrees F) for 2 hours. Then prepare it according to your pizza recipe's instructions.

5   You can freeze the dough after it has rested in the refrigerator for at least 8 hours. On a lightly floured work surface, using a sharp knife or bench scraper, divide the dough into 4 equally weighted pieces and shape them into balls. Coat each ball with olive oil and place it in its own ziplock freezer bag. The dough can be frozen for up to 3 months. To use, defrost it in the refrigerator for at least 12 hours, then let it sit at room temperature for 2 hours.

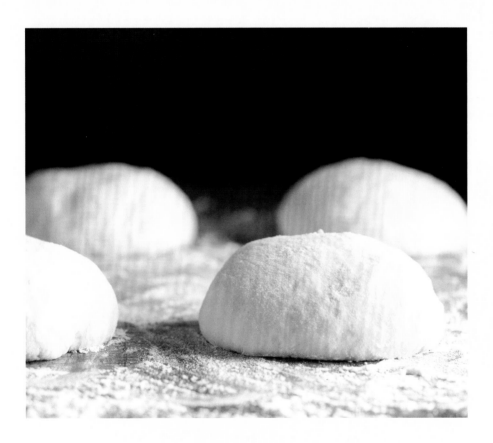

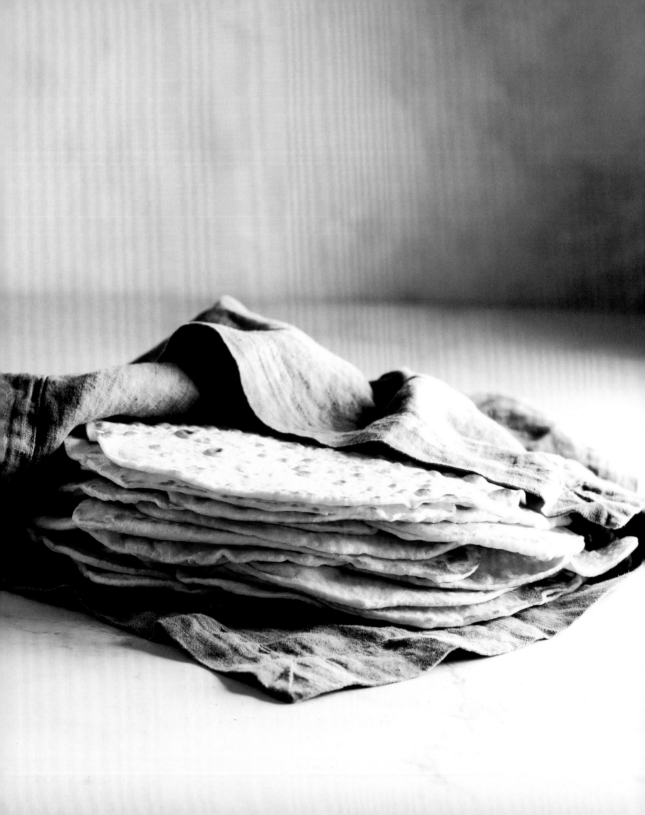

Flour Tortillas

While store-bought corn tortillas are usually very low in sodium, an 8-inch flour tortilla typically has about 130 milligrams of sodium compared to this version, which has only 32 milligrams per tortilla. The tortillas freeze really well, so you can just pull one out when needed for a burrito or wrap.

Makes: About 16 medium-size tortillas

TOTAL SODIUM: 519 mg

SODIUM PER TORTILLA:
About 32 mg

———————

4 cups (480 grams) all-purpose flour

1 tablespoon sodium-free baking powder
1 teaspoon granulated sugar
½ teaspoon light salt

¼ cup vegetable shortening, unsalted butter, or coconut oil
2 tablespoons unsalted butter
1½ cups warm water (110 degrees F)

1 Sift the flour and baking powder into a medium bowl and stir in the sugar and salt. Add the vegetable shortening and butter to the flour mixture, and, using clean fingers, work the fats into the flour until well incorporated and no large lumps remain. Add half of the water and stir with a fork to form a shaggy dough. Slowly add the remaining water until you can form a smooth dough.

2 Turn the dough out onto a lightly floured surface and knead for about 1 minute. Cover with a damp, non-terry towel and let it rest for 10 minutes. Using a sharp knife or bench scraper, divide the dough into 16 equally weighted portions, and roll each portion into a small ball. Cover with the damp towel again, and let the dough rest for at least 15 minutes and up to 1 hour.

3 When the dough has rested, heat a large cast-iron skillet or a griddle over medium-high heat until a splash of water quickly evaporates.

4 Working with 1 ball of dough at a time on a lightly floured work surface, roll the ball out into an 8-inch round thin enough that you can just start to see through the dough. Use the rolling pin to transfer the tortilla to the skillet and cook on one side until it is slightly bubbly all over, about 30 to 45 seconds. Use a spatula to flip the

continued

tortilla and cook it on the other side until browned in spots, another 30 to 45 seconds. Transfer the tortilla to a plate and cover it with a cloth to keep it warm. Repeat with the remaining dough balls.

5   Cooled tortillas can be stored in a large ziplock bag in the refrigerator for up to 4 days.

6   To freeze the tortillas for up to 6 months, layer squares of parchment paper between each tortilla, put them in a ziplock bag, and squeeze as much air out of the bag as possible before sealing. To reheat, remove from the plastic bag, wrap in aluminum foil still frozen, and bake in a preheated 350-degree-F oven for about 15 minutes.

Variation: Tortilla Chips

You can use Flour Tortillas (page 61) or store-bought corn tortillas for these low-sodium chips, which are great with Mango Salsa (page 15), Pico de Gallo (page 14), Red Chile Sauce (page 89), Green Chile Sauce (page 90), or guacamole. If using corn tortillas, first bake them at 250 degrees F for 8 minutes to dry them out, which will make them crisper when fried.

Makes: About 60 chips
TOTAL SODIUM: 324 mg (flour), 100 mg (corn)
SODIUM PER CHIP: About 5 mg (flour), about 2 mg (corn)

4 cups frying oil, such as safflower

8 to 10 tortillas

1 teaspoon citric salt (optional)

In a medium heavy-bottomed pot, heat the oil until it registers 350 degrees F on an instant-read thermometer. While the oil is heating, slice each tortilla into 6 or 8 triangles. Working with about 5 triangles at a time, use a slotted spoon to carefully lower them into the oil (it should start bubbling frantically). Fry until the bubbling calms down, about 1 minute on each side. Transfer the chips to paper towels to drain and sprinkle with a pinch of the citric salt. Repeat with the remaining triangles, keeping an eye on the oil temperature to maintain 350 degrees.

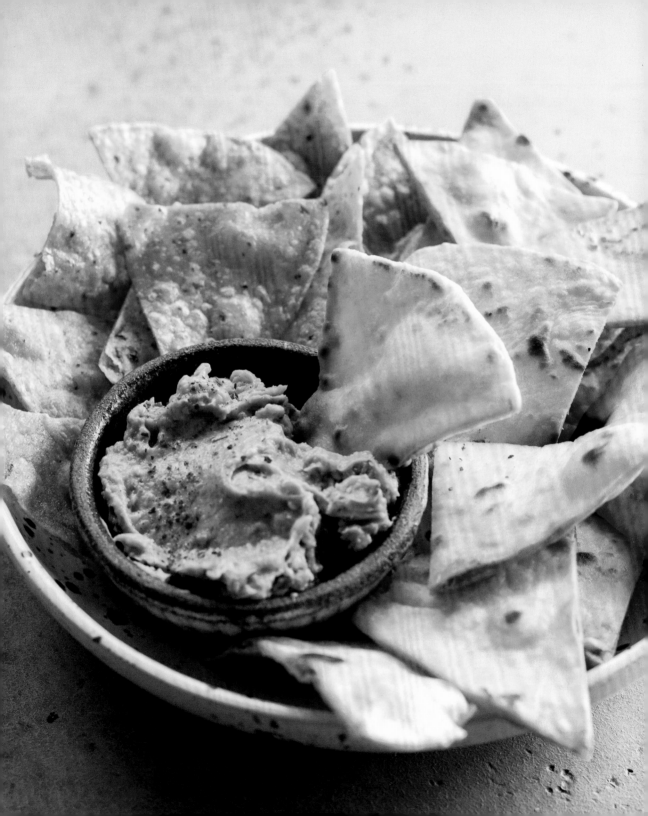

Naan

Naan is traditionally baked in a very hot wood-fired oven. Since you probably don't have one of those at home, a cast-iron skillet makes a fine substitute. Or, if you are grilling, you can throw naan on a hot grill until it is bubbly and slightly charred in spots, about a minute on each side.

Want garlic naan? Just add minced garlic to the butter when you are melting it.

Makes: 12 naan

TOTAL SODIUM: 390 mg

SODIUM PER NAAN: About 33 mg

4 cups (480 grams) bread flour

2 tablespoons granulated sugar

2 teaspoons (1 packet) active dry yeast

¼ teaspoon light salt

1 cup plain yogurt

¾ cup water at 80 degrees F

2 tablespoons unsalted butter, melted, plus more for serving

Vegetable oil, for greasing

1 In the bowl of a stand mixer fitted with the dough hook attachment, lightly whisk the flour, sugar, yeast, and salt. Add the yogurt and water, and stir until the flour is mostly moistened. Knead the dough on medium speed for 1 minute. If there is still dry flour on the bottom of the bowl, add a bit more water. Knead for an additional 4 minutes on medium-high, until the dough is smooth. Cover the bowl with plastic wrap and let it rest in a warm spot (70 to 75 degrees F) until doubled in volume, at least 1 hour.

2 Turn the dough onto a generously floured work surface. Use the heel of your (clean) hand to gently punch down the dough, then use a sharp knife or bench scraper to cut the dough into 12 equal portions. Roll each piece into a ball and arrange the balls on the work surface, leaving at least 2 inches between them. Cover with plastic wrap, then a towel. Let the dough rest until doubled in volume, about 30 minutes.

3 When you are ready to cook the naan, heat a lightly oiled cast-iron skillet over medium-high heat until hot to the touch. Place a bowl of water and a pastry brush next to your work surface. Roll or stretch one of the dough balls into an oblong about ¼ inch thick, like you would pizza dough. Lightly brush both sides with a bit of water. Place it on the hot skillet and cook until you see bubbles forming on the top side, about 1 minute. Flip the naan and cook it for another minute, pressing down on the bread if the bubbles get too big. If serving immediately, brush one side with a little bit of butter. Repeat with the remaining dough balls.

4 Cooled naan can be refrigerated in a ziplock bag for up to 4 days. Reheat it in a 350-degree-F oven and brush with butter to serve.

5 To freeze the naan for up to 6 months, layer squares of parchment paper between each one, put them in a ziplock freezer bag, and squeeze as much air out of the bag as possible before sealing. To reheat, remove from the plastic bag, wrap in aluminum foil still frozen, and bake in a preheated 350-degree oven for about 15 minutes.

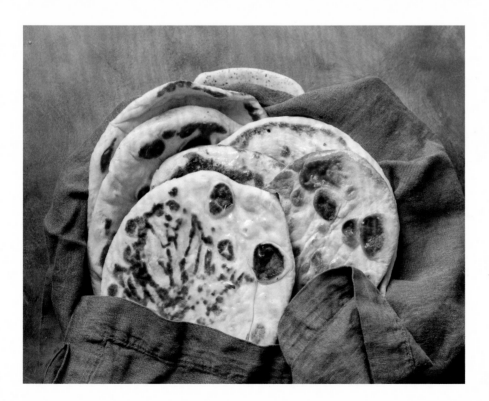

Biscuits

The key to getting super-flaky biscuits is grating the butter, which makes it easy to lightly incorporate the fat into the flour. You can use regular milk in this recipe, but buttermilk will add a bit more flavor. If you don't have buttermilk, substitute plain yogurt for up to half of the milk.

Makes: 5 large or 10 small biscuits

TOTAL SODIUM: 439 mg

SODIUM PER BISCUIT:
88 mg (large),
44 mg (small)

2½ cups (300 grams) all-purpose flour

1 tablespoon sodium-free baking powder

¼ teaspoon light salt

½ cup (1 stick) unsalted butter, well chilled

¾ cup buttermilk or whole milk

1 tablespoon apple cider vinegar

1 tablespoon cream

1 tablespoon water

1   Preheat the oven to 425 degrees F and line a baking sheet with parchment paper.

2   Sift the flour into a large bowl and stir in the baking powder and salt. Using the large holes of a cheese grater, grate the butter into the flour and toss lightly with a fork.

3   In a small bowl, mix the milk and apple cider vinegar. Pour half the milk mixture into the flour mixture, and lightly stir. Add the remaining milk, focusing on the dry areas, and stir until you have a shaggy dough. Do not overwork the dough. There may still be some dry spots. Using clean hands, fold the dough over itself in the bowl 3 or 4 times until the dry bits are incorporated.

4   Turn the dough out onto a lightly floured work surface, and lightly roll it to about 1½ inches thick. Fold the dough over itself and reroll it to 1½ inches. Repeat this 2 more times. Using a 2½- or 3½-inch biscuit cutter, cut out the biscuits to the preferred size. I use a sharp knife instead of a biscuit cutter to cut them into squares so there is no need to reroll the scraps.

5   To bake, place the biscuits on the baking sheet, leaving at least 1 inch between them. In a small bowl, mix the cream with the water to make a wash, and brush the tops of the biscuits. This will help the tops to brown. Bake until the biscuits are golden brown on top, 10 to 18 minutes (smaller biscuits should be ready in about 10 minutes). Transfer the biscuits to a wire rack to cool slightly, about 5 minutes. These are best served warm.

6   To freeze, place unbaked biscuits on a parchment-lined baking sheet and freeze until solid. Transfer the frozen biscuits to a ziplock freezer bag; they will keep, frozen, for up to 3 months. Bake the biscuits from frozen as you would from fresh—but they may need to bake a few more minutes.

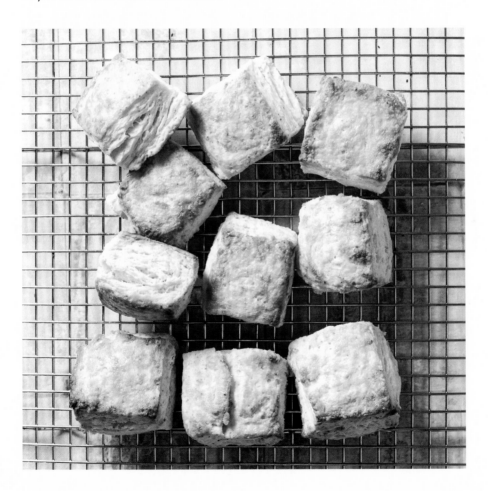

Brown Butter Sage Corn Bread

Some cornbread is completely savory, and some is basically cake with a bit of corn in it. This cornbread is somewhere in the middle. It's subtly sweet and bakes up with a slightly crisp crust, thanks to the cast-iron skillet, but inside has a tender, cakey crumb.

Makes: About 12 pieces

TOTAL SODIUM: 778 mg

SODIUM PER PIECE: About 65 mg

1½ cups (180 grams) fine yellow cornmeal

½ cup (65 grams) whole wheat flour

½ cup (60 grams) all-purpose flour

1½ tablespoons sodium-free baking powder

1 teaspoon sodium-free baking soda

½ teaspoon dried sage

¼ teaspoon light salt

¾ cup (1½ sticks) unsalted butter, cut into pieces

2¼ cups whole milk

½ cup honey

3 large eggs

½ cup fresh or frozen corn (optional)

1   Preheat the oven to 375 degrees F.

2   In a medium bowl, whisk together the cornmeal, whole wheat and all-purpose flours, baking powder, baking soda, sage, and salt. Set aside.

3   In a large 10-inch cast-iron skillet over medium heat, melt the butter, and swirl to coat the sides of the pan. Continue to cook, stirring frequently, until the foam subsides, the butter is a medium golden brown, and the solids have separated and turned a toasty brown, about 10 minutes. Be careful not to burn the butter; reduce the heat if it's browning too quickly.

4   Transfer the brown butter to a large bowl and add the milk and honey, whisking until the mixture is smooth and has cooled, about 2 minutes. Whisk in the eggs. Pour the mixture into the cornmeal mixture, add the corn, and gently stir to combine.

5   Heat the empty skillet in the oven for 2 minutes, then carefully scrape the batter into the hot skillet. Bake until the top is browned around the edges and a skewer inserted into the center comes out clean, 25 to 35 minutes.

6   Allow the cornbread to cool in the pan for at least 10 minutes before slicing and serving. Wrap any leftover cornbread in plastic wrap and store at room temperature for up to 2 days.

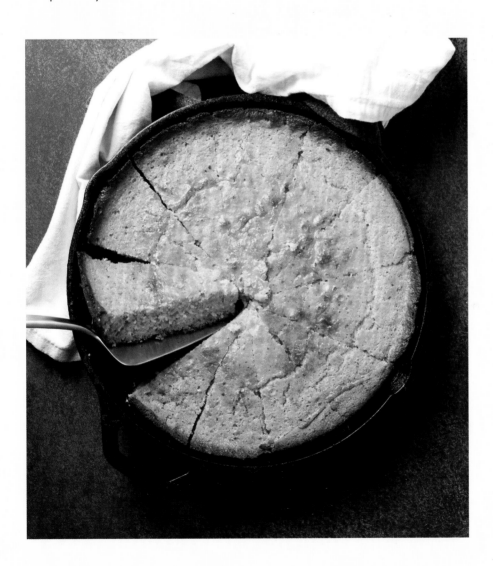

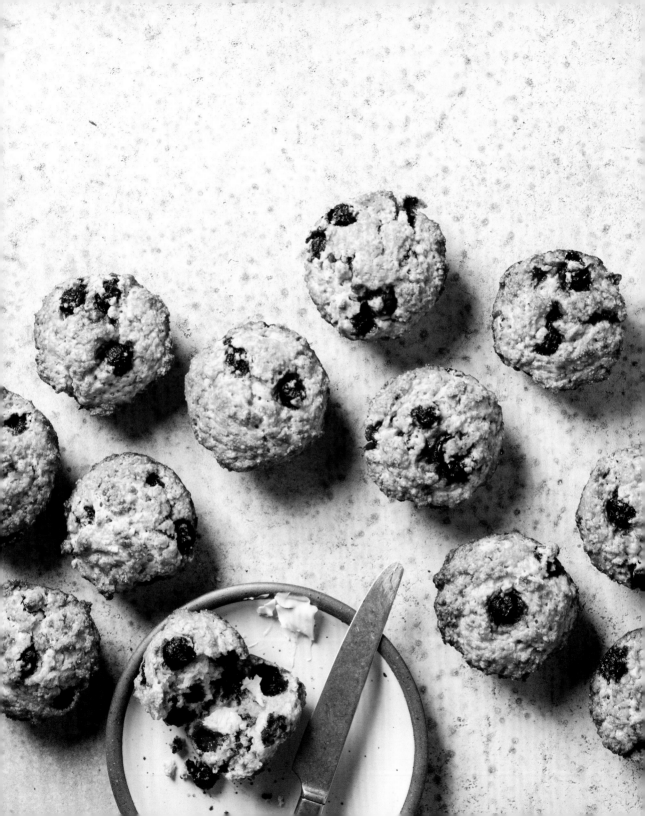

Mix-In Muffins or Quick Bread

I believe that muffins should not be breakfast cupcakes. To me, they should be just barely sweet and have a rustic texture and just enough crumb to hold together the fruit. This recipe does the trick and also bakes up well as a quick bread.

Makes: 12 standard muffins or 1 loaf

TOTAL SODIUM: 534 mg (without mix-ins)

SODIUM PER MUFFIN OR SLICE: About 45 mg

2½ cups (300 grams) all-purpose flour

⅓ cup granulated sugar, plus more for sprinkling

¼ cup lightly packed light or dark brown sugar

1 tablespoon sodium-free baking powder

¼ teaspoon light salt

2 large eggs

½ cup yogurt or sour cream

½ cup whole milk or buttermilk

1 teaspoon vanilla extract

½ cup (1 stick) unsalted butter, melted

Mix-ins (see page 72)

1   To make muffins, preheat the oven to 375 degrees F. Lightly grease a 12-cup muffin tin with vegetable oil, or line the tin with paper liners.

2   In a medium bowl, whisk together the flour, both sugars, baking powder, and salt. Gently stir in the mix-ins you are using.

3   In a large bowl, whisk together the eggs, yogurt, milk, and vanilla. Stir in the flour mixture and melted butter. It's OK if some lumps remain.

4   Divide the batter equally among the muffin cups. If you'd like, sprinkle the tops of the muffins with a pinch of granulated sugar.

5   Bake until the muffins are light brown and a skewer inserted into the center of a muffin comes out clean, 30 to 40 minutes. Let the muffins cool in the tin for 5 minutes, then cool on a wire rack for about 15 minutes.

continued

6   Once they have cooled completely, the muffins can be frozen. Reheat from frozen, wrapping the muffins in aluminum foil and baking at 350 degrees F for about 10 minutes.

7   To make quick bread, spoon the batter into a lightly oiled 8½-by-4½-by-3-inch loaf pan and sprinkle the top with a pinch of granulated sugar if desired. Bake at 350 degrees F until the top of the loaf is a deep golden brown and a skewer inserted into the center comes out clean, 50 to 60 minutes. Allow the loaf to cool in the pan on a wire rack for 10 minutes, then invert the pan to remove the loaf. It's best to let the loaf cool completely before cutting.

Mix-Ins

Here are some great options to try:

- 1½ cups frozen or fresh blueberries + zest of 1 medium lemon
- 1½ cups frozen or fresh cranberries + zest of 1 medium orange + ½ cup chopped unsalted toasted walnuts
- 1½ cups frozen or fresh raspberries + ½ cup chopped unsalted toasted pecans
- 1 cup frozen or fresh diced peaches + 1 teaspoon cinnamon + ½ cup chopped unsalted toasted pecans
- 1 cup dried cherries (soaked and drained) + ½ cup chopped unsalted toasted almonds
- ¾ cup fresh diced plums + 1 teaspoon ground allspice
- ½ cup chopped pistachios + 1 teaspoon ground cardamom
- 1 cup dried apricots (soaked and drained) + ½ cup chopped unsalted toasted walnuts

Pie Dough

I learned the basics of this recipe from the "piechiatrist" herself, Kate McDermott, James Beard Award–nominated author of *Art of the Pie*. Although her recipe can be made as is without the salt, it is then really bland. I like my pie crust to have a little flavor, and by using a little light salt, sugar, and a splash of vinegar, you get a pie crust worth nibbling on even without any filling.

Makes: Enough dough for 1 double pie crust

TOTAL SODIUM: 285 mg

SODIUM PER SLICE: About 36 mg

2½ cups (300 grams) all-purpose flour

1 tablespoon granulated sugar

¼ teaspoon light salt

14 tablespoons chilled unsalted butter, cut into pieces

2 tablespoons apple cider vinegar

⅓ cup ice water

1   Sift the flour, sugar, and salt into a medium bowl, and whisk together. Using clean hands, work the butter into the flour until there are no clumps bigger than a pea.

2   In a small bowl, mix the vinegar and water. Add it to the flour mixture 2 tablespoons at a time, mixing between each addition with a fork, until the dough starts to come together. Then use your hands to form it into a ball.

3   Divide the dough in half, and press each half into a disc about 1 inch thick. Wrap each disc tightly in plastic wrap and refrigerate for at least 1 hour before using. You can also freeze the dough at this point and defrost it in the refrigerator before using.

"Box" Yellow Cake Mix

My husband's favorite cake is from a box, and I still married him. As someone who loves to bake from scratch, I jokingly judge him for it, but I can't really blame him. Boxed cake mix is really easy and predictable, and I'll admit, it makes a pretty fluffy cake. Of course, like most chemically leavened baked goods, there is too much sodium in the mix, so I created this "box" version that is just as easy. Every year for his birthday, I use it to bake him Duncan Hines–esque devil's food cupcakes.

To make chocolate cake mix, substitute ½ cup (60 grams) of the flour with Dutch-process cocoa powder.

Makes: About 5 cups dry mix (enough for 1 cake or 18 cupcakes)

TOTAL SODIUM: 418 mg

2½ cups (300 grams) cake flour or all-purpose flour

1¾ cups granulated sugar

⅓ cup dry milk powder

1½ tablespoons sodium-free baking powder

½ teaspoon sodium-free baking soda

¼ teaspoon light salt

1   In a large bowl, whisk all the ingredients together. Store in an airtight container at room temperature for up to 1 month or in the freezer for up to 3 months.

Yellow Cake

Makes: 1 cake or 18 cupcakes

TOTAL SODIUM: 564 mg

TOTAL PER SERVING:
  About 47 mg per
  slice or 31 mg per
  cupcake (unfrosted)

1 recipe "Box" Yellow
  Cake Mix (see
  opposite page)
1 cup water

2 large eggs
¼ cup vegetable oil
½ teaspoon vanilla
  extract

Preheat the oven to 325 degrees F. Lightly grease your preferred baking pan with vegetable oil, or line two 12-cup muffin pans with 18 cupcake liners. To make the cake, in a large bowl, combine all the ingredients and beat for 2 minutes or until smooth. Pour the batter into the prepared pan(s). Bake until lightly golden and a skewer inserted into the center comes out clean.

PAN SIZE	BAKE TIME
9-by-13-inch rectangle	34 to 38 minutes
Two 8-inch round	32 to 36 minutes
10-inch (6- to 8-cup) fluted tube	35 to 40 minutes
18 cupcakes	16 to 20 minutes

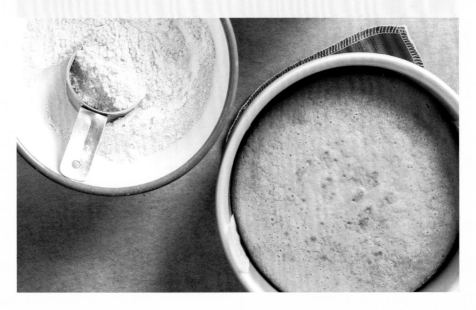

Stocks, Beans & Sauces

Chicken Stock

Though it's a little cheaper to buy chicken stock, it won't be nearly as delicious as this. Be sure to save the meat from the wings after you make the stock: you can use it to easily pull together soups or stews, such as my Chicken & Rice Stew (page 155). I recommend using only the drumette and wingette portions: the tips don't have much meat, but they do have a lot of small bones, which are tricky to pick out.

Makes: 8 cups
TOTAL SODIUM: 866 mg
SODIUM PER CUP: About
   108 mg

2 pounds chicken wings
1 medium onion, diced

½ cup diced carrot
   (about 1 medium)
2 cloves garlic, crushed
1 bay leaf
¼ cup loosely packed
   fresh flat-leaf parsley
   leaves

1 tablespoon fresh thyme
   leaves
1 tablespoon black
   peppercorns
1 tablespoon apple cider
   vinegar
8 cups water

1   If you are using a multicooker, put all the ingredients in the pot. Cover, being sure to set the steam vent to closed. Cook on high pressure for 30 minutes, then let the stock sit on low heat for at least 20 minutes and, for the richest stock, up to 2 hours to naturally release. Carefully open the steam vent according to the manufacturer's instructions.

2   If you are cooking the stock on the stovetop, put all the ingredients in a medium stockpot over medium-high heat and bring to a simmer. Reduce the heat to medium and continue to simmer until the liquid is reduced by about one-third, about 90 minutes. There's no need to bother with skimming.

3   Strain the stock through a fine-mesh sieve and allow it to cool before storing. If you are saving the meat, carefully pull the wings from the sieve and set them aside to cool. When they are cool enough to handle, remove the bones (they should pull out easily, leaving the meat).

4   Refrigerate the stock in an airtight container for up to 5 days or freeze for up to 6 months: divide the cooled stock into portions and pour it into freezer bags. Thaw in the refrigerator before using.

Beef Stock

Bone broth has been having a bit of a moment, but it's really just long-simmered beef stock made with bones that have lots of collagen— look for oxtails, neck bones, or any sort of knuckle. You may be able to get them really inexpensively if you have a local butcher. If you can't find them, use short ribs.

For an even richer, darker broth, roast the bones for thirty minutes at 450 degrees F before following the steps below.

Makes: 8 cups
TOTAL SODIUM: 775 mg
SODIUM PER CUP: About
   97 mg

---

3 pounds assorted beef
   bones
1 medium onion, diced
½ cup diced carrot
   (about 1 medium)
4 cloves garlic, crushed
1 bay leaf
¼ cup loosely packed
   fresh flat-leaf parsley
   leaves
¼ cup dried mushrooms
1 tablespoon fresh thyme
   leaves
1 tablespoon black
   peppercorns
1 tablespoon apple cider
   vinegar
8 cups water

1   If you are using a multicooker, put all the ingredients in the pot. Cover, being sure to set the steam vent to closed. Cook on high pressure for 45 minutes, then let the stock sit on low heat for at least 20 minutes and, for the richest stock, up to 2 hours to naturally release. Carefully open the steam vent according to the manufacturer's instructions.

2   If you are cooking the stock on the stovetop, put all the ingredients in a small stockpot over medium-high heat and bring to a simmer. Reduce the heat to medium and continue to simmer until the stock is a deep golden color, about 12 to 14 hours.

3   Strain the stock through a fine-mesh sieve and allow it to cool before storing.

4   Refrigerate the stock in an airtight container for up to 5 days or freeze for up to 6 months: divide the cooled stock into portions and pour it into freezer bags. Thaw in the refrigerator before using.

Vegetable Broth

This rich vegetable broth has a delicious flavor worthy of stirring into risotto, using as a base for a favorite soup, or even sipping on its own.

Makes: 12 cups
TOTAL SODIUM: 195 mg
SODIUM PER CUP: About
  16 mg

---

2 celery ribs, diced
1 medium onion, diced
1 apple, halved
½ cup diced carrot
  (about 1 medium)
½ cup dried shiitake
  mushrooms

1 sheet nori
3 tablespoons nutritional
  yeast flakes
3 cloves garlic, crushed
2 dried bay leaves
¼ cup loosely packed
  fresh flat-leaf parsley
  leaves
1 tablespoon fresh thyme
  leaves

½ tablespoon black
  peppercorns
1 teaspoon fennel seed
1 teaspoon coriander
  seed
2 tablespoons olive oil
1 tablespoon apple cider
  vinegar
1 tablespoon tomato
  paste
12 cups water

1   If you are using a multicooker, put all the ingredients in the pot. Cover, being sure to set the steam vent to closed. Cook on high pressure for 25 minutes, then let the stock sit on low for another 10 minutes. Carefully quick-release the steam vent according to the manufacturer's instructions.

2   If you are cooking the broth on the stovetop, put all the ingredients in a small stockpot over medium-high heat and bring to a simmer. Reduce the heat to medium and continue to simmer until the broth is a deep golden color, about 50 minutes.

3   Strain the broth through a fine-mesh sieve and allow it to cool before storing.

4   Refrigerate the broth in an airtight container for up to 5 days or freeze for up to 6 months: divide the cooled broth into portions and pour it into freezer bags. Thaw in the refrigerator before using.

Thick-Skinned Beans

Using dried beans instead of canned not only saves you sodium, it saves you money. This basic recipe works for any kind of thick-skinned beans, such as kidney, pinto, great northern, cranberry (also called borlotti), and cannellini. If you have a multicooker, your total cooking time will be less than an hour.

It's been a long-standing food debate whether beans cooked with salted water made a "creamier" bean or not. If you are on the pro-salted-water side, you could add ¼ teaspoon light salt to the water when soaking and cooking. I've tried it both ways, and in my experience, a bit of salt does help prevent some bean bursting in the cooking process, but to me, it's not worth the added sodium. I'd rather save my sodium for seasoning the finished dish.

Makes: About 6 cups cooked beans

TOTAL SODIUM: 88 mg, depending on bean type

SODIUM PER CUP: About 15 mg, depending on bean type

2 cups dried kidney, pinto, or other thick-skinned beans

1   Rinse the beans well under cool water, removing any small stones or other detritus that might be lurking.

2   Now you have a choice: to soak or not to soak. If you have time, soaking the beans will help them better retain their shape and reduce cooking time. To soak the beans: Put them in a large bowl and cover with at least 2 inches of water. Let them soak for at least 12 hours and up to 30 hours, adding more water if needed. Once the beans have soaked, drain them in a colander and rinse well.

3 If you are using a multicooker, put the beans in the pot and add enough water to cover them by about 2 inches. Cover, being sure to set the steam vent to closed. If you've soaked the beans, cook on high pressure for 10 minutes for firm beans or 15 minutes for very soft beans. For unsoaked beans, cook on high pressure for 40 minutes for firm beans or 50 minutes for very soft beans. Let the cooker naturally release without opening the pressure valve. Then carefully open the steam vent according to the manufacturer's instructions.

4 If you are cooking the beans on the stovetop, put them in a large, heavy-bottomed pot. Add enough water to cover them by at least 3 inches and bring to a simmer over medium-high heat. Cover and simmer, stirring occasionally, until the beans have softened to the desired consistency, 2 to 4 hours.

5 To refrigerate for up to 5 days: Put the beans in an airtight container and add enough cooking liquid to just cover them. To freeze for up to 6 months: Allow the beans to cool completely. Drain them in a colander, then transfer them to freezer bags. Defrost overnight in the refrigerator before using.

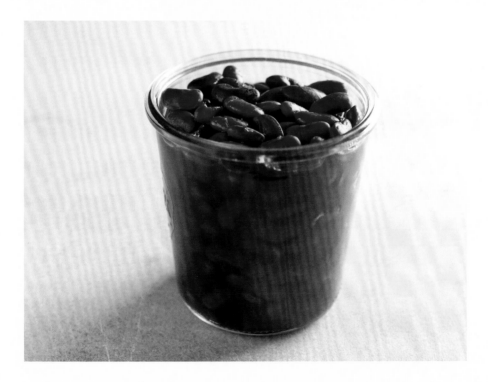

Chickpeas

Chickpeas (also called garbanzo beans) are great for throwing into salads, pastas, or of course, making Hummus (page 110). Like other beans, starting from dried instead of canned ensures they are low in sodium.

Your cooking time may vary based on the beans and how you are using them; if you are cooking them on the stovetop, you'll want to first soak them eight hours to overnight. If you are using a multicooker, cooking time may vary based on the make and model; if the beans are not the desired texture after the natural release, just repressurize and continue to cook them, for ten minutes at a time, until you get the right texture. If you want the beans for a stew that will continue to cook, keep them firmer. For hummus, you'll want them quite soft.

If you want to save the liquid (called aquafaba) to use as an egg substitute, soak your beans overnight before cooking them even if you are using a pressure cooker. You may also need to reduce the aquafaba in a pot over low heat if it is too thin; it should be somewhat syrupy. The aquafaba will keep, refrigerated, for about three days.

Makes: About 6 cups cooked beans

TOTAL SODIUM: 96 mg   SODIUM PER CUP: About   2 cups dried chickpeas
                             16 mg

1   Rinse the beans well under cool water, removing any small stones or other detritus that might be lurking.

2   If you are using a multicooker, put the beans in the pot and add enough water to cover them by about 2 inches. Cover, being sure to set the steam vent to closed. Cook on high pressure for 35 minutes for firm beans and 50 minutes for very soft beans. Let the cooker naturally release without opening the pressure valve. Then carefully open the steam vent according to the manufacturer's instructions.

3   If you are cooking the beans on the stovetop, put them in a large, heavy-bottomed pot. Add enough water to cover them by 3 inches and bring to a simmer over medium-high heat. Cover and simmer, stirring occasionally, until the beans have softened to the desired consistency, 2 to 3 hours.

4   To refrigerate for up to 5 days: Put the beans in an airtight container and add enough cooking liquid to just cover them. To freeze for up to 6 months: Allow the beans to cool completely. Drain them in a colander, then transfer them to freezer bags. Defrost overnight in the refrigerator before using.

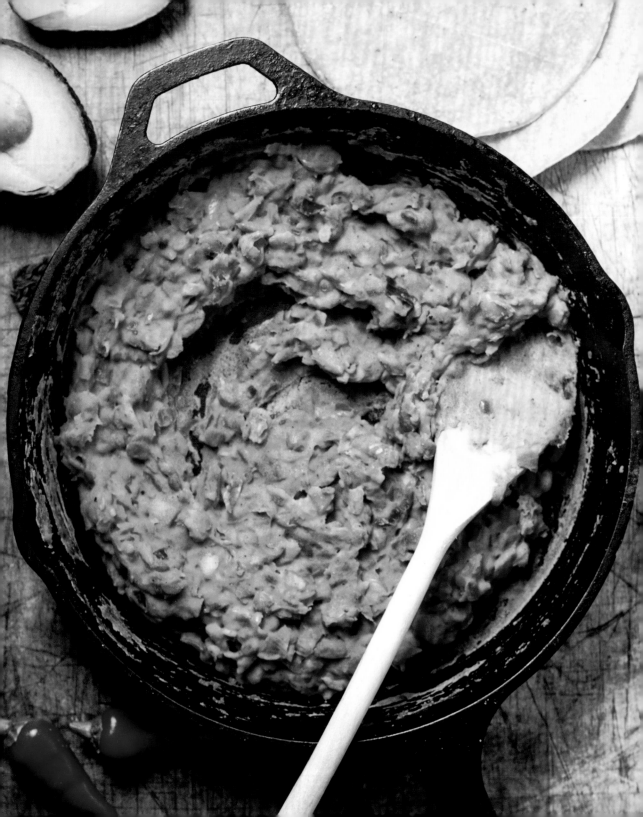

Refried Beans

While refried beans are traditionally made with pinto beans, you can make them with just about any variety. I like them with black beans, in particular, but also try them with great northern beans, black-eyed peas, or cranberry beans. A pile of beans, a couple of eggs, and a healthy swirl of red or green chile sauce on top is a great meal any time of the day.

This recipe starts with softly cooked beans, but if you haven't already done that, I recommend tossing half an onion and a clove or two of garlic into the pot when cooking the dried beans for even more flavor.

Makes: About 2 cups

TOTAL SODIUM: 305 mg

SODIUM PER CUP: About 153 mg

2 tablespoons olive oil
½ medium onion, chopped
2 cloves garlic, minced
½ teaspoon cumin seeds
½ teaspoon dried oregano
½ teaspoon freshly ground black pepper
¼ teaspoon cayenne or chipotle pepper
¼ teaspoon light salt
2 cups pinto beans (see page 80)

1   In a large skillet, heat the oil over medium-high heat until it is shimmering. Reduce the heat to low and add the onion. Cook until softened, about 5 minutes. Add the garlic, cumin seeds, oregano, black pepper, cayenne pepper, and salt, and cook until fragrant, another 5 minutes. Stir in the beans and about ½ cup of either the liquid from the beans or water. Use the back of a wooden spoon to gently mash the beans to the desired texture. (If you want completely smooth beans, you can use an immersion blender.) Taste and season with a bit more black pepper if needed.

2   Refrigerate the beans in an airtight container for up to 5 days. To freeze cooked beans for up to 6 months, allow them to cool completely, then spoon them into freezer bags. Defrost overnight in the refrigerator before using.

Black Beans

Unlike kidney beans and other thicker-skinned beans, black beans are better cooked without a presoak. Also, I find that aromatics greatly enhance the flavor of black beans.

Makes: About 6 cups cooked beans

TOTAL SODIUM: 54 mg

SODIUM PER CUP: About 9 mg

2 cups dried black beans

1 tablespoon olive oil (optional)

1 bay leaf (optional)

1 medium onion, halved and skin removed (optional)

2 cloves garlic (optional)

1   Rinse the beans well under cool water, removing any small stones or other detritus that might be lurking.

2   If you are using a multicooker, put all the ingredients in the pot and add enough water to cover them by about 2 inches. Cover, being sure to set the steam vent to closed. Cook on high pressure for 20 minutes for firm beans and 25 minutes for very soft beans. Let the cooker naturally release without opening the pressure valve. Then carefully open the steam vent according to the manufacturer's instructions.

3   If you are cooking the beans on the stovetop, put all the ingredients in a large, heavy-bottomed pot. Add enough water to cover them by 3 inches and bring to a simmer over medium-high heat. Cover and simmer, stirring occasionally, until the beans have softened to the desired consistency, 2 to 4 hours.

4   To refrigerate for up to 5 days: Put the beans in an airtight container and add enough cooking liquid to just cover them. To freeze for up to 6 months: Allow the beans to cool completely. Drain them in a colander, then transfer them to freezer bags. Defrost overnight in the refrigerator before using.

Pomodoro (Tomato) Sauce

This recipe, based on Marcella Hazan's most famous sauce, makes plenty for a pound of cooked pasta, but you might consider making a double or triple batch and freezing the excess to whip up a quick weeknight pasta without much effort. Toss in some Beef & Pork Meatballs (page 93) for an even heartier treat. You'll want to use about 1½ cups of sauce per pound of pasta.

Makes: About 2 cups
TOTAL SODIUM: 53 mg
SODIUM PER CUP: About
27 mg

1 (28-ounce) can unsalted peeled whole or chopped tomatoes
5 tablespoons unsalted butter

1 medium onion, halved
¼ cup chopped fresh basil (optional)
1 tablespoon balsamic vinegar

1   In a medium heavy-bottomed saucepan over medium heat, simmer all the ingredients, stirring occasionally, until thickened to your liking, 30 to 45 minutes. Use the back of a wooden spoon to break up any large tomato pieces.

2   Refrigerate the sauce in an airtight container for up to 5 days. To freeze for up to 6 months, allow the sauce to cool completely, then spoon it into freezer bags. Thaw overnight in the refrigerator before using.

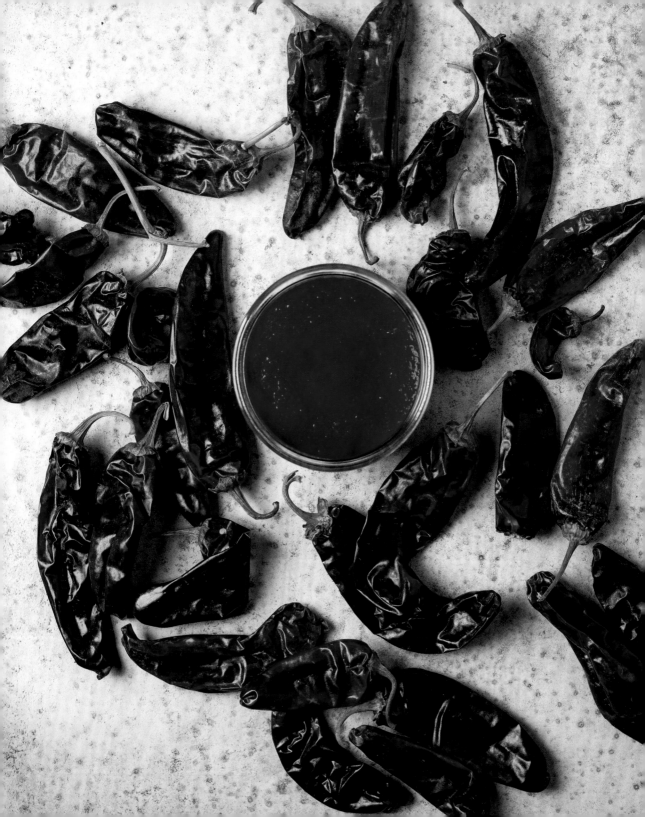

Red Chile Sauce

A large part of my family lives in New Mexico, so I typically use New Mexico red chilies in this sauce, which is great for enchiladas, huevos rancheros, wet burritos, or stewed meats. You can substitute any large dried red chilies, such as guajillo, ancho, or pasilla.

Makes: About 3 cups
TOTAL SODIUM: 450 mg
SODIUM PER CUP: About
150 mg

10 to 12 dried New Mexico red chilies or other dried red chili peppers, stemmed, seeded, and torn into rough pieces

1 clove garlic
½ cup chopped yellow onion
1 tablespoon olive oil
½ cup water
1 cup Chicken Stock (page 77)

½ teaspoon ground cumin
½ teaspoon dried oregano
¼ teaspoon light salt

1   Put the chilies in a large saucepan with enough water to cover them and bring to a boil over medium heat. Reduce the heat, and simmer for 5 minutes. Remove the pan from the heat and allow the chilies to cool to room temperature.

2   When the chilies have cooled, remove them with a slotted spoon and transfer to a blender or the bowl of a food processor. Add the garlic, onion, oil, and the water. Blend until smooth, adding a bit more water if the sauce is too thick.

3   Strain through a fine-mesh sieve to remove any remaining bits of chili and return to the saucepan over medium heat. Stir in the chicken stock, cumin, oregano, and salt, and simmer until thickened, about 20 minutes.

4   Refrigerate sauce in an airtight container for up to 5 days. To freeze for up to 6 months, allow the sauce to cool completely, and then spoon it into freezer bags. Thaw overnight in the refrigerator before using.

Green Chile Sauce

Try to find fire-roasted New Mexico green chilies (like Hatch) for this recipe for the best flavor. If you can't locate any, it's fine to use frozen or even canned green chilies. I prefer frozen—which you can order from quite a few places online, and usually don't have any added salt—but if you do use canned, make sure it's just the chilies.

I'll also often use fresh Anaheim chilies and roast them myself under the broiler. Don't skip the roasting step: it's important to the flavor.

Makes: About 2 cups
TOTAL SODIUM: 253 mg
SODIUM PER CUP: About 127 mg

1 tablespoon olive oil
½ cup chopped onion

1 pound fire-roasted green chilies, chopped
1 clove garlic, minced
2 teaspoons all-purpose flour

1 cup Chicken Stock (page 77)
⅛ teaspoon light salt
Freshly ground black pepper

1   Heat the oil in a large cast-iron skillet over medium-low heat. When the oil is hot, add the onion and cook until softened, about 10 minutes. Add the chilies and garlic and sauté until softened, another 3 minutes. Stir in the flour and add the stock a little at a time, stirring well between each addition. Simmer until thickened, about 20 minutes, then stir in the salt. Season to taste with black pepper.

2   Refrigerate the sauce in an airtight container for up to 5 days. To freeze for up to 6 months, allow the sauce to cool completely, then spoon it into freezer bags. Thaw overnight in the refrigerator before using.

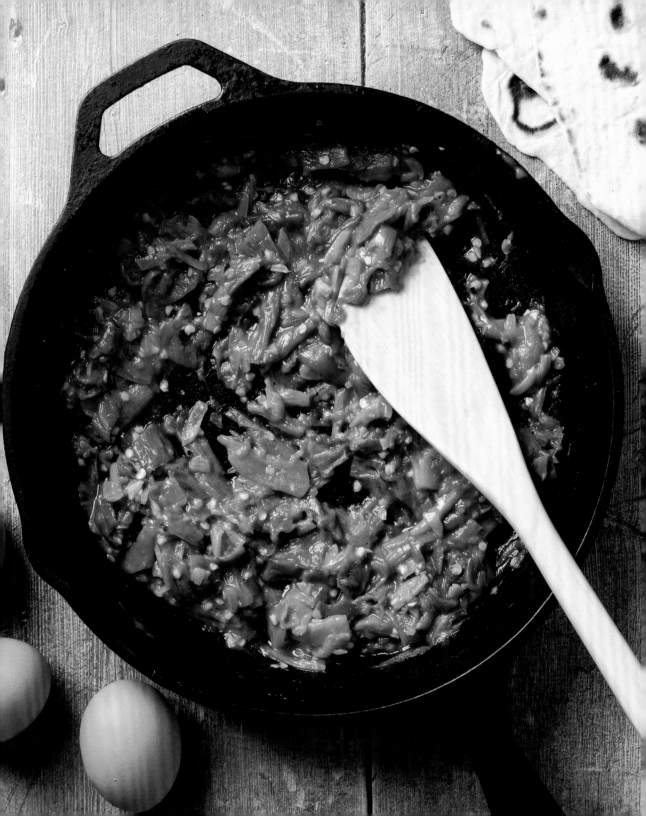

Meats, Cheeses & Spreads

Beef & Pork Meatballs

You can pan-fry these meatballs before baking them, but when you're making a large batch, that can be both time consuming and messy. Instead, I like to skip the frying and simply bake them, with a blast at the end under the broiler to brown them up. Make sure to use a broiler tray or rack, so the fat that would be rendered off in the frying pan doesn't congeal around the bottoms of the meatballs while they bake.

Makes: About 30 meatballs

TOTAL SODIUM: 1,167 mg
SODIUM PER MEATBALL:
   About 39 mg

———————

1 pound ground beef
1 pound ground pork
2 large eggs

1 clove garlic, minced
¼ cup grated Parmesan
2 tablespoons chopped
   fresh flat-leaf parsley
   leaves
1 teaspoon dried oregano

½ teaspoon freshly
   ground black pepper
Pinch of red pepper
   flakes
1½ cups bread crumbs
   (see page 52)
¾ cup water

1   Preheat the oven to 400 degrees F.

2   In a large bowl, using clean hands, combine the beef and pork. Add the eggs, garlic, Parmesan, parsley, oregano, black pepper, and red pepper flakes, and mix well. Add the bread crumbs and mix thoroughly. Add the water a little at a time and continue to mix until all the water has been added. Form the mixture into 2½-inch balls and place on a broiler pan or a 13-by-18-inch rack placed atop a baking sheet.

3   Bake the meatballs until cooked through, 20 to 25 minutes. Turn on the broiler and broil until the tops are browned, about 5 minutes.

4   Serve immediately, or allow to cool to room temperature before storing. The meatballs can be refrigerated in an airtight container for up to 5 days. To freeze, line a baking sheet with parchment paper, then place the meatballs on the baking sheet and freeze for 30 minutes. Transfer them to freezer bags and store in the freezer for up to 4 months.

Italian Sausage

Italian sausage has a lot of flavor, but often a lot of that flavor is salt. This sausage packs a punch from fennel seed, smoked paprika, and garlic, and I don't think you'll miss the salt at all. It's a terrific pizza topping (such as for Italian Sausage & Mushroom Pizza on page 171) and is also great mixed with the Pomodoro (Tomato) Sauce (page 87) on pasta.

Makes: 2 pounds (32 ounces)

TOTAL SODIUM: 766 mg

SODIUM PER OUNCE:
About 24 mg

2 pounds ground pork

2 teaspoons crushed garlic

2 teaspoons fennel seeds, lightly crushed

1 teaspoon freshly ground black pepper

1 teaspoon cayenne pepper (optional)

1 teaspoon smoked paprika

1 teaspoon red pepper flakes (optional)

¼ teaspoon light salt

1   In a large bowl, thoroughly combine all the ingredients. Put the uncooked sausage in an airtight container and refrigerate overnight or for up to 5 days to let the flavors meld.

2   At this point, you can either cook the sausage or freeze it in bulk. To freeze, divide the sausage into four ½-pound portions, then wrap each one tightly in plastic wrap. Store in the freezer for up to 4 months. Defrost for 8 hours in the refrigerator before using.

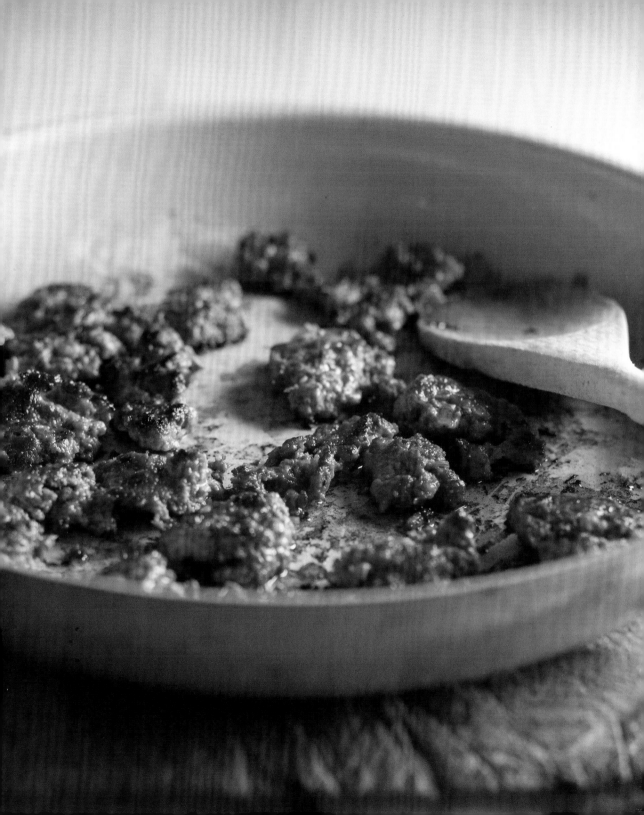

Breakfast Sausage Patties

A glug of maple syrup gives this sausage just a hint of sweetness. Form it into patties and make a breakfast sandwich by pairing it with an egg on a biscuit. These patties freeze well, and there's no need to defrost them—simply cook them from frozen for a quick breakfast.

Makes: 2 pounds (32 ounces)

TOTAL SODIUM: 765 mg

SODIUM PER OUNCE:
About 24 mg

2 pounds ground pork

2 tablespoons maple syrup

1 teaspoon fennel seeds, lightly crushed

1 teaspoon dried sage

1 teaspoon freshly ground black pepper

1 teaspoon smoked paprika

½ teaspoon garlic powder

½ teaspoon dried thyme

¼ teaspoon light salt

⅛ teaspoon freshly grated nutmeg

1   In a large bowl, thoroughly combine all the ingredients. Put the uncooked sausage in an airtight container and refrigerate overnight or for up to 3 days to let the flavors meld.

2   At this point, you can either form the breakfast patties or freeze the sausage in bulk. To form, scoop ¼ cup of sausage, roll it into a ball, and smash the ball into a ¼-inch-thick patty. Repeat with the remaining sausage. To freeze, divide the sausage into four ½-pound portions, then wrap each one tightly in plastic wrap. Store in the freezer for up to 4 months. Defrost for 8 hours in the refrigerator before using.

3   Once the patties are formed, in a large cast-iron skillet over medium-high heat, cook them in batches, being careful not to overcrowd the pan, until browned and cooked through, about 2 minutes on each side.

4   You can refrigerate the cooled patties in an airtight container for up to 5 days or freeze them for up to 4 months. To freeze, line a baking sheet with parchment paper. Place the patties on the baking sheet and freeze for 30 minutes, then transfer them to an airtight container. When reheating, fry or grill the frozen patties for 3 to 4 minutes on each side.

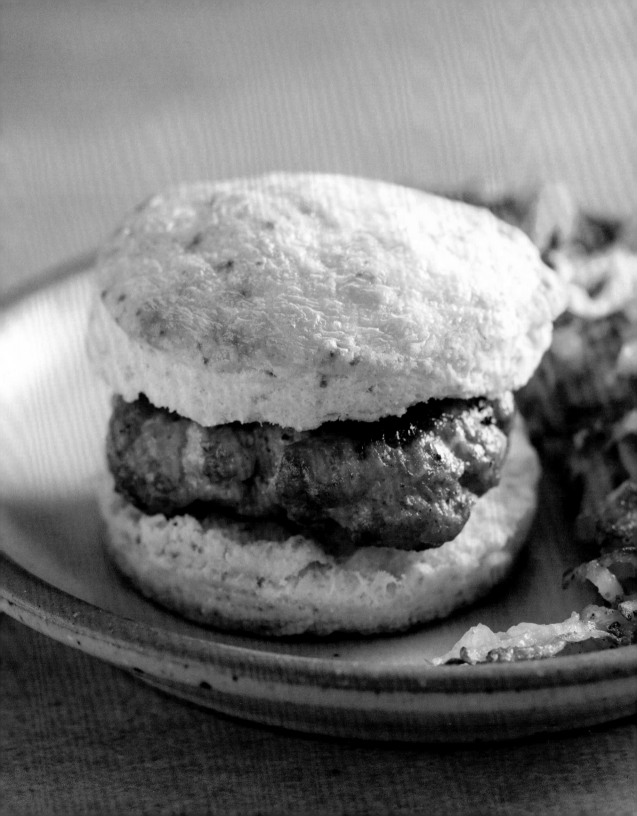

Bacon

Here's a spin on a homemade low-sodium bacon technique I learned from Jessica Goldman Foung's *Sodium Girl* blog. It slow-cooks seasoned strips of pork belly instead of using the traditional cure-and-smoke method. I'm not going to lie to you: this bacon is definitely more meaty and significantly less salty than the traditional kind. I wouldn't try to pass it off as bacon to my salt-indulging friends. But if your palate has already adjusted to low-sodium foods, your breakfast and club sandwiches can get back to bacon-y goodness.

If possible, ask your butcher to slice the pork belly for you and remove the skin. You'll want slices about ⅛ inch thick for traditional bacon or ¼ inch thick for thick-cut bacon.

If you are slicing the pork belly yourself, remove the skin and wrap the pork tightly in plastic wrap. Freeze it for one hour per pound until it firms up but is not completely frozen. Then use a very sharp knife to slice it to the desired thickness while it's still chilled.

Make about 10 slices

TOTAL SODIUM: 415 mg
SODIUM PER SLICE: About 41 mg

2 tablespoons maple syrup

1 tablespoon liquid smoke

1 tablespoon coconut aminos

1 pound pork belly, skinned and sliced

¼ teaspoon freshly ground black pepper

1   In a small bowl, combine the maple syrup, liquid smoke, coconut aminos, and pepper. Put the pork belly in a gallon-size ziplock bag and pour the maple syrup mixture over it. Seal the bag and shake it to coat each of the slices. Refrigerate for at least 1 hour and up to 12 hours (longer is better, as more of the seasoning can permeate the meat).

2 Preheat the oven to 200 degrees F. Line two baking sheets with aluminum foil, and top each with a wire rack.

3 Place the bacon strips on the wire rack, leaving about ½ inch between each slice. Bake for 1 hour, until the meat has darkened and some of the fat has rendered. *Note: This just parcooks the bacon. It still needs to be fried or otherwise cooked before eating.* At this point, you can cook the bacon or allow it to cool completely before storing it.

4 Wrap the cooled, unfried bacon in plastic wrap and refrigerate in an airtight container for up to 5 days. Or layer it on wax paper, wrap the wax paper tightly in plastic wrap, and freeze for up to 4 months. Defrost overnight in the refrigerator before frying.

5 Fry the bacon as you would store-bought bacon, being careful not to overcrowd the pan. Transfer to a paper towel to drain.

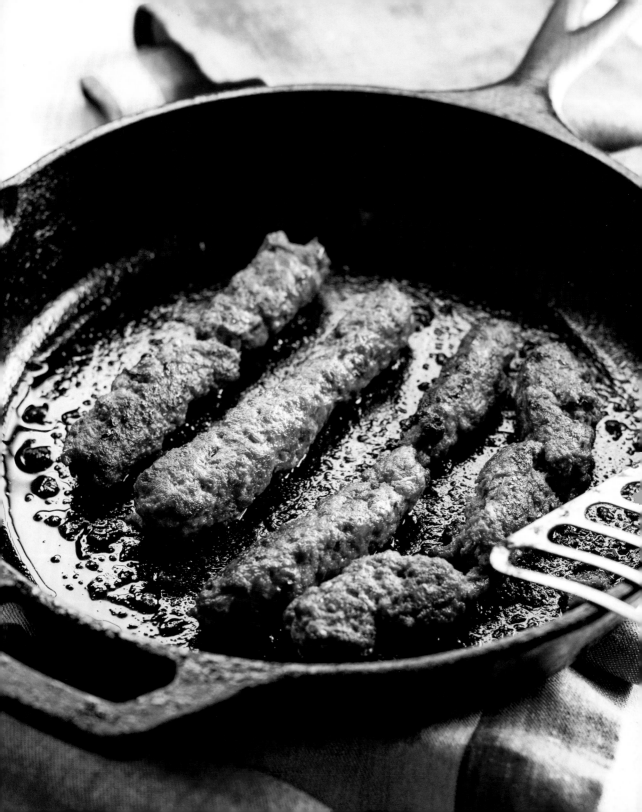

Merguez

Merguez is a North African lamb (or sometimes beef) sausage spiked with harissa. It's typically served in a casing, but this recipe skips that step. With a little bit of care, you can form it into the shape you want, such as patties, and grill it without the casing, or just keep it in bulk. Merguez also makes great meatballs!

Makes: About 2 pounds (32 ounces)

TOTAL SODIUM: 917 mg

SODIUM PER OUNCE:
  About 29 mg

___

1 teaspoon coriander seeds

1 teaspoon cumin seeds

1 teaspoon fennel seeds

½ teaspoon ground cinnamon

½ teaspoon ground turmeric

¼ teaspoon cayenne pepper

2 pounds ground lamb

4 cloves garlic, minced

3 tablespoons Harissa (page 8)

2 tablespoons tomato paste

2 tablespoons chopped fresh cilantro leaves

2 teaspoons grated fresh ginger

¼ teaspoon light salt

1   In a small skillet over medium-low heat, toast the coriander, cumin, and fennel seeds until fragrant, about 1 minute. Transfer to a spice grinder or a mortar, along with the cinnamon, turmeric, and cayenne pepper, and finely grind.

2   Put the lamb in a large bowl, along with the ground spices, garlic, harissa, tomato paste, cilantro, ginger, and salt. Use clean hands to knead the mixture and mix well. (You can also do this in the bowl of a stand mixer fitted with the paddle attachment.)

3   Form the mixture into whatever shape you want. Refrigerate the sausage in an airtight container for up to 5 days or freeze for up to 4 months wrapped tightly in plastic wrap. Defrost in the refrigerator before using.

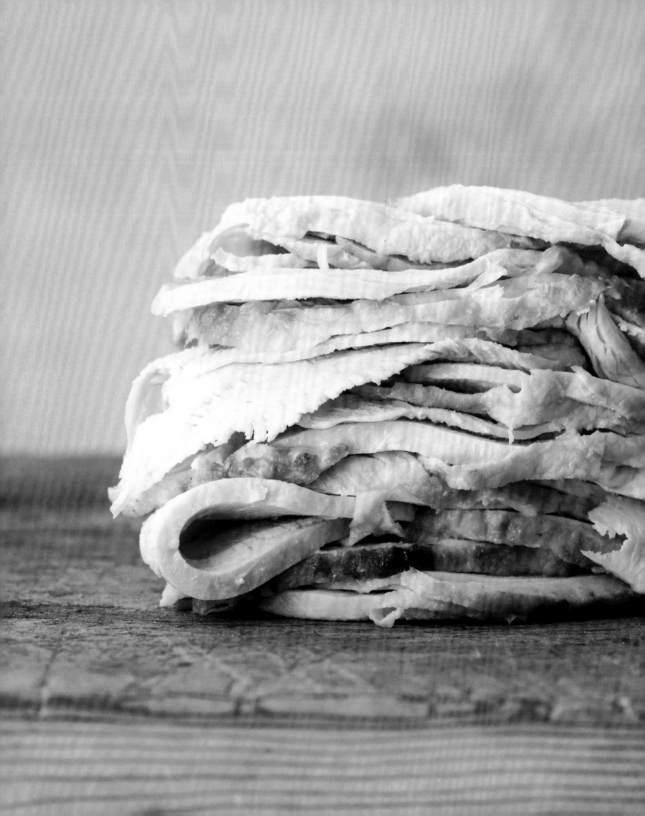

Roasted Turkey Lunch Meat

Store-bought deli turkey meat typically contains more than 350 milligrams of sodium per two-ounce serving. While you may be able to find low-sodium turkey in some markets, it's actually quite easy to make your own, and you can cut it as you'd like—sliced thin or thick for sandwiches, or cubed for salads. Using a multicooker that can accommodate a turkey breast will make especially quick work of it.

Makes: 40 (2-ounce) servings

TOTAL SODIUM: 1,900 mg

SODIUM PER SERVING:
   About 48 mg

———————

⅓ cup maple syrup

2 tablespoons coconut aminos

1 tablespoon lemon zest

2 teaspoons liquid smoke

½ teaspoon fresh thyme leaves

½ teaspoon citric acid

½ teaspoon freshly ground black pepper

5 pounds uncooked turkey breast

1 cup white wine

1   In a large bowl, combine the maple syrup, coconut aminos, lemon zest, liquid smoke, thyme, citric acid, and pepper. Place the turkey breast in the bowl. Use your fingers to gently release the skin from the top of the turkey breast. Using clean hands, smear about half of the mixture under the skin, spreading evenly. Then use the rest to coat the skin. If your turkey breast is skinless, just spread the whole mixture evenly over the top. Cover the bowl with plastic wrap, or, if it fits, place the turkey with marinade in a large ziplock bag, and refrigerate for at least 2 hours and up to 12 hours (the longer you marinate it, the better the flavor).

2   Preheat the oven to 175 degrees F.

3   Place the turkey breast on a rack in a deep roasting pan (if the breast has been cut, place the cut side down). Pour the wine into the bottom of the roasting pan.

4   Roast the turkey until an instant-read thermometer inserted into the thickest part of the breast registers 165 degrees F, about 4 hours.

continued

5   If you are using a multicooker, place the turkey breast on a rack in the pot. Cover, being sure to set the steam vent to closed. Cook on high pressure for 27 minutes. Let the cooker naturally release without opening the pressure valve. Then carefully open the steam vent according to the manufacturer's instructions.

6   To brown the skin afterward, broil in the oven for about 5 minutes.

7   When the turkey breast has cooked, remove it from the oven, tent with aluminum foil, and let it rest until it comes to room temperature. Slice it to the desired thickness.

8   Refrigerate in an airtight container or wrapped in plastic wrap for up to 5 days, or divide it into 1- to 2-pound batches, wrap them well in plastic wrap, and freeze for up to 4 months. Defrost in the refrigerator before using.

Ricotta

Ricotta is the perfect "starter cheese" if you've never made cheese before. It's as simple as heating milk, adding a bit of acid, and then scooping out and draining the fresh cheese curds. Spread it on toast, topped with a spoonful of Blistered Cherry Tomatoes (page 206) or a drizzle of honey, or dollop a spoonful on a bowl of pasta.

Be sure to use fresh, pasteurized milk for any cheese-making. Ultra-pasteurized milk does not form curds well.

Makes: About 2 cups cheese and 5 cups whey

TOTAL SODIUM (CHEESE):
  400 mg
SODIUM PER TABLESPOON
  (CHEESE): About 13 mg

½ gallon whole milk
¼ teaspoon light salt

⅓ cup freshly squeezed lemon juice (from 2 medium lemons)

1   Line a fine-mesh sieve with a double layer of cheesecloth, and place it over a medium bowl.

2   Rinse a medium saucepan with cold water, which will help prevent scorching, and add the milk and salt. Simmer over medium-low heat until the milk registers 185 degrees F on an instant-read thermometer, about 15 minutes. Reduce the heat to low and stir in the lemon juice. If curds don't form after 2 minutes, add another 1 to 2 tablespoons of lemon juice. Continue to simmer as the curds firm, and the remaining whey becomes clear, about 10 minutes.

3   Using a slotted spoon, carefully scoop the curds into the sieve, reserving the whey. Let the curds drain, undisturbed, for about 10 minutes, or until cool, then transfer them to an airtight container. Refrigerate and use within 2 days.

4   Use the reserved whey to cook pasta or brine pork chops for pan-searing. If you don't need the whey immediately, you can freeze it in an airtight container or freezer bag for up to 4 months.

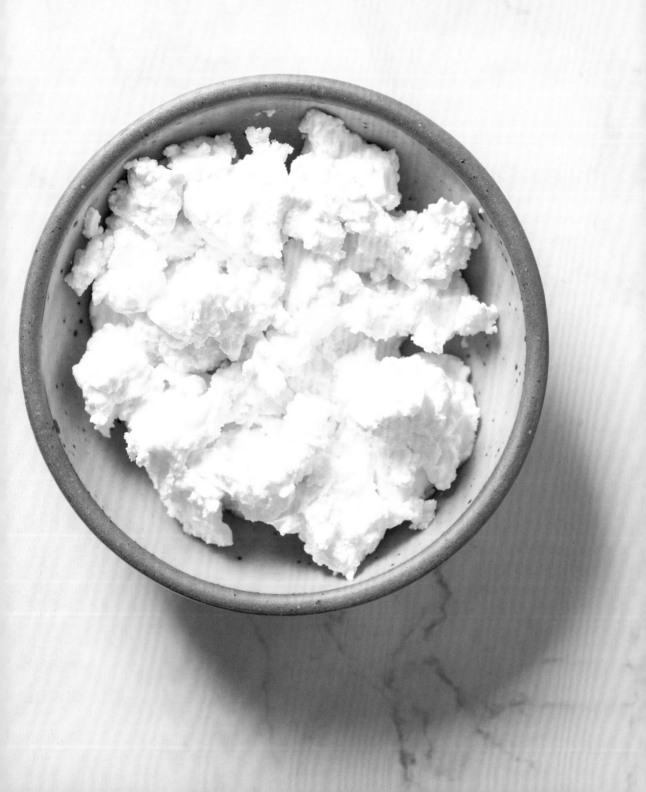

Chèvre (Fresh Goat Cheese)

While you probably won't find chèvre starter in your local grocery store, it's easily found online: Amazon carries it, or you can order directly from the New England Cheesemaking Supply Company or Cultures for Health.

Pasteurized goat milk, on the other hand, may be harder to find. Most grocery stores only carry ultra-pasteurized goat milk, which doesn't work well for cheese-making. However, with a little searching, you can usually find a farm nearby that offers it as part of a dairy delivery service. In Washington, DC, I get mine from South Mountain Creamery, and it is well worth seeking out.

The curds will need to drain for up to twelve hours, so find a corner of your kitchen where they can sit undisturbed. If you have a Greek yogurt strainer, this is a great time to use it. A muslin-lined tofu press also works great.

Makes: About 1½ cups

TOTAL SODIUM: 586 mg

SODIUM PER TABLESPOON: About 24 mg

½ gallon pasteurized goat milk

Chèvre starter (follow the manufacturer's instructions regarding quantity)

1   Rinse a medium nonreactive saucepan with cold water, which helps prevent scorching, and add the milk. Simmer over low heat until the milk registers 86 degrees F on an instant-read thermometer, about 3 minutes. Turn off the heat and sprinkle the starter on top. Let the starter sit for about 1 minute, then stir it into the milk.

2   Cover the pan with a towel and let the milk sit at room temperature (ideally around 72 degrees F) until it thickens, about 12 hours. The curds won't look quite like cow's milk curds, but they'll thicken to the texture of a Greek yogurt.

continued

3   Line a fine-mesh sieve with cheesecloth, leaving enough overhang to create a bag when the ends are gathered. Set the sieve over a bowl. Using a slotted spoon, carefully scoop the curds into the sieve, discarding the whey, and let them drain for about 10 minutes. Then grab the edges of the muslin and tie them together. Slip the handle of a wooden spoon or other stick through the tied portion of the muslin and hang the cheese over a deep bowl or bucket so that it continues to drain.

4   Let the curds drain at room temperature for up to 12 hours, depending on the consistency you'd like. For a softer, smoother cheese, drain for only a couple of hours. For firmer cheese that you can use as crumbles, let them drain the full 12 hours.

5   Refrigerate the cheese, well wrapped in plastic wrap, for up to 1 week or freeze for up to 2 months. Defrost in the refrigerator before using. Frozen goat cheese is best used in recipes where the goat cheese is whipped in.

Variation: Marinated Goat Cheese

Makes: ½ cup

TOTAL SODIUM: 200 mg

SODIUM PER TABLESPOON:
   About 25 mg

4 ounces Chèvre
¼ cup olive oil
2 (3-inch) strips fresh
   orange zest

2 small fresh bay leaves
1 clove garlic, smashed
1 whole star anise pod,
   or 2 whole cloves
½ teaspoon coriander
   seeds, crushed

¼ teaspoon red pepper
   flakes
2 tablespoons chopped
   fresh herbs, such as
   cilantro, parsley, or
   dill, for garnish

Cut rounds of firm goat cheese, or dollop soft goat cheese into a shallow bowl. In a small saucepan over very low heat, warm the oil, zest, bay leaves, garlic, star anise, coriander seeds, and red pepper flakes, stirring frequently until the garlic begins to brown, about 5 minutes. Take the pan off the heat and let cool for at least 10 minutes. Pour the oil mixture over the goat cheese and let it sit at room temperature for at least 30 minutes and up to 3 hours. Pluck out and discard the zest, bay leaves, garlic, and anise pod, and garnish the cheese with the fresh herbs. Spread the cheese on toasted baguette slices, bagels, or pita chips, or dollop in a salad. Refrigerate the cheese, covered, for up to 2 weeks.

Cream Cheese

There are different methods for making cream cheese. Cultured cream cheese uses a probiotic starter and is made similar to yogurt, with a long wait. Fresh cream cheese uses an acid to separate the curds from the whey, like making ricotta. Both cheeses are great for smearing on your bagel, but I usually choose the fresh version because it involves minimal preplanning.

Cream cheese curds aren't as defined as other cheeses, such as ricotta, and because of the cream, which doesn't curdle as easily, its whey won't be as clear, so I don't usually reuse the whey from this recipe.

Makes: About 1½ cups
TOTAL SODIUM: 200 mg
SODIUM PER TABLESPOON:
   About 8 mg
_____

1 pint heavy cream
1 pint whole milk
2 tablespoons buttermilk
¼ teaspoon light salt

¼ cup distilled white vinegar or freshly squeezed lemon juice

1   Line a fine-mesh sieve with a double layer of cheesecloth, and place it over a medium bowl.

2   Rinse a small saucepan with cold water, which helps prevent scorching, and add the cream, milk, buttermilk, and salt. Simmer over medium-low heat until the milk registers 185 degrees F on an instant-read thermometer, about 15 minutes. Reduce the heat to low and stir in the vinegar. Continue to simmer as the curds firm. The mixture won't separate as much as if you were making ricotta, but the whey will slightly clear after about 5 minutes.

3   Using a slotted spoon, carefully scoop the curds into the sieve, discarding the whey. Let the curds drain, undisturbed, until cool. Stir them with a wooden spoon until the cheese is combined and smooth, or use a whisk to whip them for lighter cream cheese before storing in an airtight container in the refrigerator. Use within 2 days.

Hummus

Hummus is a great snack to have on hand to enjoy with crudités or spread on a bagel. You can jazz it up with additions such as a cup of cooked sweet potato, a smashed medium avocado, or a chopped jalapeño half. Sometimes I leave the salt out entirely, for a virtually sodium-free dip.

For the smoothest hummus, remove the skins from the chickpeas before blending. They should easily slide off. However, even if you skip this step, the hummus will be delicious.

Makes: About 2 cups
TOTAL SODIUM: 271 mg
SODIUM PER TABLESPOON: About 8 mg

———————

1 cup cooked Chickpeas (page 82)
2 cloves garlic
Juice of 2 medium lemons

3 tablespoons tahini
1 tablespoon olive oil, plus more for garnish
½ teaspoon ground turmeric (optional)
½ teaspoon *amchoor* powder (optional)
¼ teaspoon light salt

Sumac, red pepper flakes, smoked paprika, or Za'atar (page 41), for garnish
Chopped parsley, cilantro, or basil, for garnish

1   Drain the chickpeas in a colander and reserve the liquid.

2   Transfer the chickpeas to the bowl of a food processor and puree until smooth. If the mixture is too thick, add 1 tablespoon of the reserved liquid (or water, if you don't have any reserved liquid) at a time until you get a smooth puree. Add the garlic, about two-thirds of the lemon juice, and tahini, along with any additions you are using. Pulse until combined, 2 to 3 minutes. Add the oil, turmeric, *amchoor*, and salt, and pulse to combine. Taste and add a bit more lemon juice if needed.

3   Scoop the hummus into a serving dish, garnish with the spices and herbs, and drizzle a little more olive oil over the top.

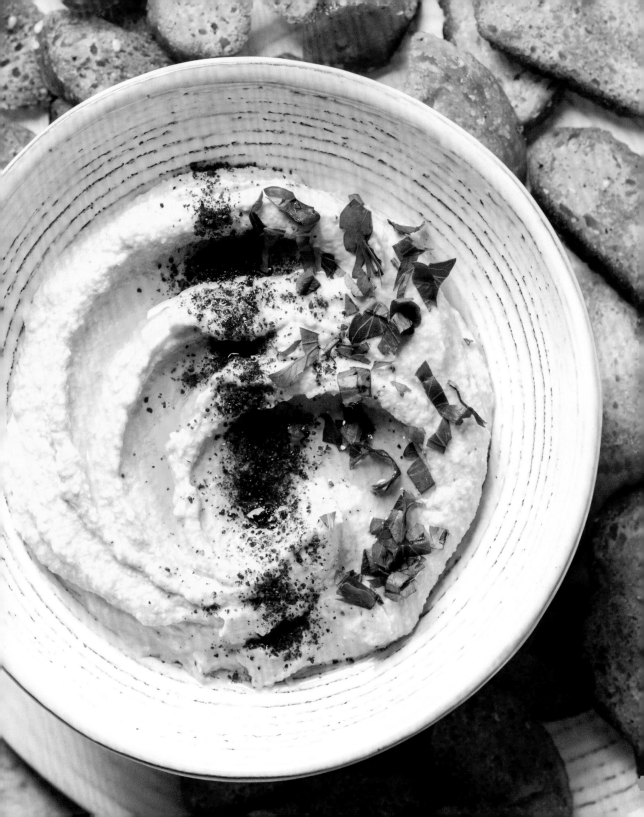

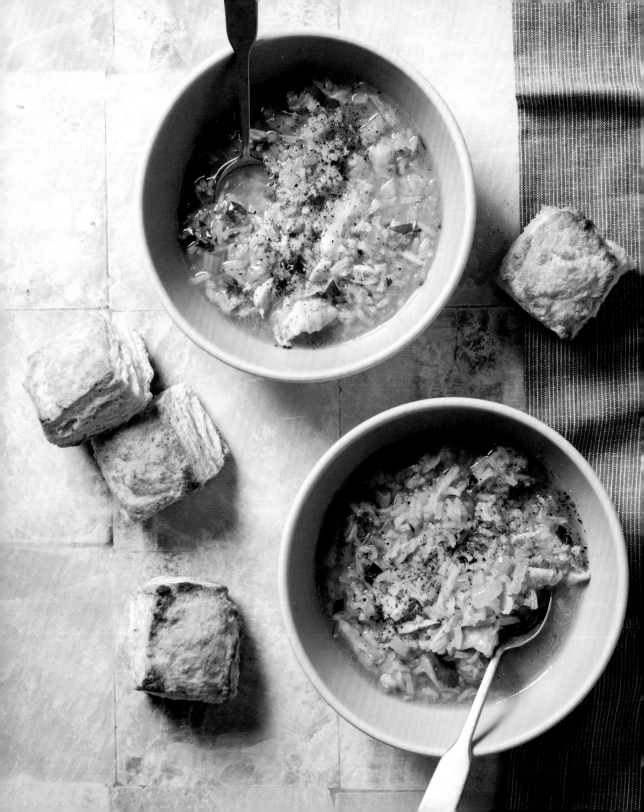

PART II:

RECIPES FOR DAILY MEALS

I get a daily email from the *New York Times* with suggestions about what to eat, and it motivates me to get into the kitchen to cook something (even if it's not what they say I should cook). That's what I hope the recipes in this section do for you. These dishes can be paired together to make a whole meal plan for the day while staying within a total sodium budget of 1,400 to 1,800 milligrams. Pick a breakfast, something light for lunch, a main course, a few sides, and even dessert: most contain less than 200 milligrams of sodium per serving. I've included some of my all-time favorite dishes, as well as plenty of options for weeknights that come together quickly and meals you can serve when celebrating. Use these recipes as a starting point to learn the basics of low-sodium cooking and then make them your own, or take the techniques (and your low-sodium staples) and adapt other recipes that inspire you.

Breakfast

Yeasted Waffles

During our last move, I knew I was moving into a smaller kitchen, so I purged a lot of my appliances, including my waffle iron. I don't know what I was thinking—a waffle iron really doesn't take up much space, but it brings so much joy! I soon remedied my mistake with an inexpensive Belgian waffle iron.

This batter, based on a recipe from Serious Eats, not only works great for Belgian waffles, but also in a standard waffle iron. Note that you'll get a few more waffles with a non-Belgian iron.

These waffles require that you rest the batter overnight, so be sure to plan ahead. But they also freeze well, so I recommend making a double batch and freezing the remainder for toaster waffles later.

Makes: Five 6½-inch Belgian-style waffles

TOTAL SODIUM: 477 mg
SODIUM PER WAFFLE:
About 95 mg
—
¾ cup (1½ sticks) unsalted butter

¼ cup granulated sugar
2½ cups whole milk
2 large eggs
3 cups (360 grams) all-purpose flour

2 teaspoons active dry yeast
½ teaspoon sodium-free baking soda
Vegetable oil, for greasing (optional)

1   In a large saucepan over medium heat, melt the butter. When the butter has foamed (or turned golden brown, if you want brown-butter waffles), take the pan off the heat and stir in the sugar and milk. Whisk in the eggs. Add the flour and stir until smooth. Stir in the yeast and baking soda.

2   Transfer the batter to a bowl that is at least twice the volume of the batter, which will rise significantly overnight, and cover with plastic wrap. Do not use a container with a lid, as pressure will build up as the dough rests, and you don't want to wake up to batter exploded all over your fridge (true story). Refrigerate overnight, for at least 12 hours and up to 36 hours.

3   Follow the instructions on your waffle iron to cook the waffles.

continued

4 To freeze leftover waffles: Allow the waffles to cool to room temperature. Line a baking sheet with parchment paper. Lay the waffles in a single layer on the baking sheet, and freeze, uncovered, for 20 minutes. Stack the waffles, with squares of parchment or wax paper between each, and put them in a freezer bag, removing as much of the air as possible.

5 To reheat frozen waffles: Preheat the oven to 375 degrees F, put the frozen waffles on a baking sheet, and bake for 8 to 10 minutes, or simply pop them in a toaster.

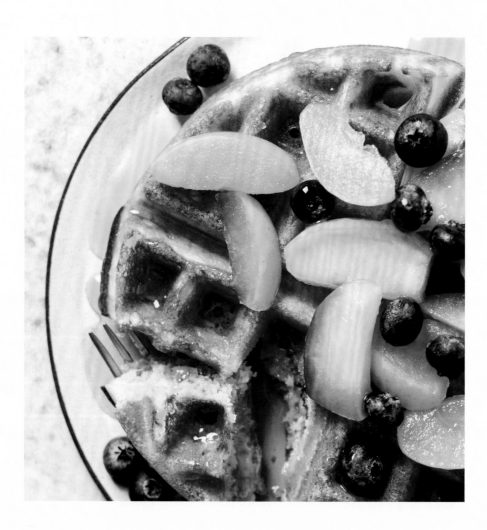

Pancakes

For breakfast, brunch, or even breakfast for dinner, a good pancake recipe is essential. This low-sodium version doesn't sacrifice any flavor or lightness. Whipping the egg whites does mean one more dirty bowl, but these pancakes are really fluffy because of it, so it's worth the extra cleanup. Add berries or bite-size pieces of fruit to make them even better.

Makes: About 15 pancakes

TOTAL SODIUM: 455 mg

SODIUM PER PANCAKE:
   About 30 mg

———————

2 cups (240 grams)
   all-purpose flour

1 tablespoon granulated
   sugar
1 teaspoon sodium-free
   baking powder
1 teaspoon sodium-free
   baking soda

2 large eggs, separated
1½ cups whole milk
1 cup yogurt
¼ cup unsalted butter,
   melted

1   In a medium bowl, mix the flour, sugar, baking powder, and baking soda.

2   In another medium bowl, whisk the egg whites until soft peaks form. Set aside.

3   In a large bowl, whisk the egg yolks, milk, and yogurt until smooth. Slowly stir in the butter. Using a rubber spatula, fold in the egg whites. Then fold in half of the flour mixture, followed by the remaining flour mixture. Do not overmix; there may still be some lumps.

4   Heat a griddle or nonstick frying pan over medium heat until it is hot to the touch. Scoop ¼ cup of the batter and pour it onto the griddle or pan. Top the pancake with any berries or other mix-ins you are using, gently pushing them into the batter. Cook until bubbles form evenly across the top, about 2 minutes, then flip with a spatula and cook until the pancake is golden brown, another 2 minutes. Repeat with the remaining batter.

continued

5   To freeze leftover pancakes: Allow the pancakes to cool to room temperature. Line a baking sheet with parchment paper. Lay the pancakes in a single layer on the baking sheet, and freeze, uncovered, for 20 minutes. Stack the pancakes, with squares of parchment or wax paper between each, and put them in a freezer bag, removing as much of the air as possible.

6   To reheat frozen pancakes: Preheat the oven to 375 degrees F, put the frozen pancakes on a baking sheet, and bake for 8 to 10 minutes.

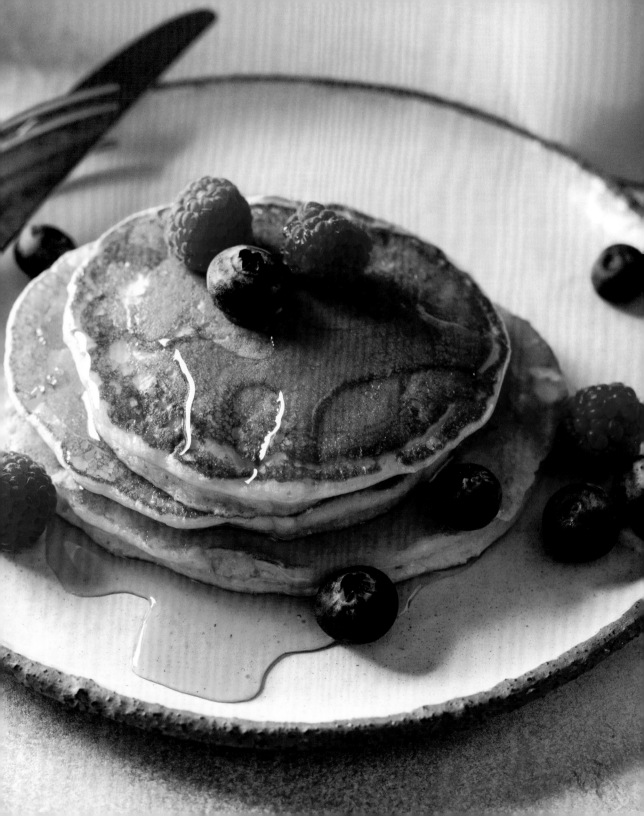

Baked Apple & Blueberry Oatmeal

I ate a lot of oatmeal when I was first diagnosed with Ménière's disease, because it was easy to make it low sodium, but although I like oatmeal porridge, it does get rather tiresome. This baked oatmeal, on the other hand, is a treat any day.

I've used apples and blueberries in this recipe, but try substituting other fruits and berries. Cranberries and oranges make a great combination in winter, or strawberry and rhubarb in spring. I use steel-cut oats, which have a firmer texture, but rolled oats work great too.

Makes: About 8 servings

TOTAL SODIUM: 563 mg

SODIUM PER SERVING:
About 71 mg

1½ cups steel-cut oats, or 3 cups rolled oats (not quick-cooking)

1 cup slivered almonds

2 teaspoons ground cinnamon

¼ teaspoon ground allspice

4 cups whole milk

¼ cup honey

2 tablespoons unsalted butter, melted, plus more for greasing

1 large egg

1 teaspoon vanilla extract

1 apple, cored and chopped

1½ cups blueberries

1 Preheat the oven to 350 degrees F and lightly grease a small ceramic baking dish.

2 In a large bowl, mix the oats, almonds, cinnamon, and allspice.

3 In medium bowl, whisk the milk, honey, butter, egg, and vanilla. Pour the milk mixture over the oat mixture and mix well. Stir in the apple and blueberries. Pour into the prepared baking dish.

4 Bake until the top is golden, and the liquid is absorbed, 40 to 50 minutes. Allow to cool for about 10 minutes before serving.

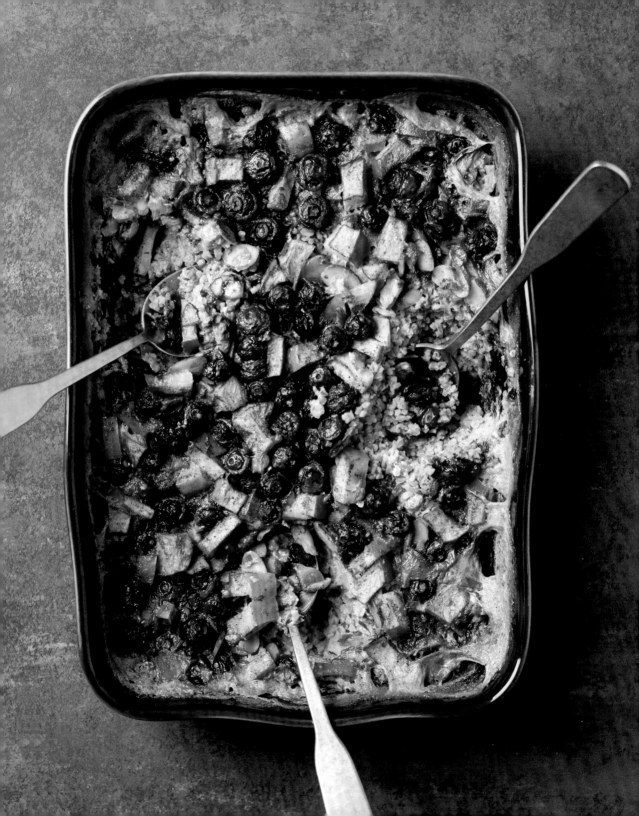

Banana Bread

Several years ago, I shot a banana bread recipe for Epicurious, and it became my go-to banana bread. When I first started on a low-sodium diet, I had some friends over, and I made this version of that recipe so I could have something to snack on while everyone else was munching down on cheese and crackers. Not realizing it was low sodium, my friends devoured it—even those that claimed that they didn't like banana bread! And it's been a request ever since.

A lot of banana breads load up on mix-ins such as nuts or chocolate chips. If that's what you like, by all means, add away. But also give it a shot the simple way. I think you'll be pleasantly surprised.

Makes: 1 loaf (about 12 servings)

TOTAL SODIUM: 365 mg

TOTAL PER SERVING:
About 30 mg

1⅔ cups (200 grams) all-purpose flour

1 teaspoon sodium-free baking powder

1 teaspoon sodium-free baking soda

½ teaspoon ground allspice

¼ teaspoon light salt

½ cup (1 stick) unsalted butter, at room temperature, plus more for greasing

⅓ cup lightly packed light brown sugar

⅓ cup granulated sugar

1 large egg

1 cup mashed ripe banana (from 2 large or 3 medium bananas)

3 tablespoons plain yogurt or sour cream

Zest of 1 medium lemon

1 teaspoon vanilla extract

1   Preheat the oven to 350 degrees F and lightly grease an 8½-by-4½-by-3-inch loaf pan.

2   In a small bowl, whisk together the flour, baking powder, baking soda, allspice, and salt.

3   In the bowl of a stand mixer, mix the butter and the sugars on medium speed until well creamed, about 5 minutes. Add the egg, banana, yogurt, zest, and vanilla, and beat on medium-high until smooth. If your ingredients are cold, the mixture may look curdled. That's OK. Add the flour mixture and mix on low until just incorporated (do not overmix).

4   Spoon the mixture into the pan and smooth the top. Bake until deep golden brown and a skewer inserted into the center comes out clean, 45 to 50 minutes. Allow the loaf to cool in the pan on a wire rack for 10 minutes, then invert the pan to remove the loaf. It's best to let the loaf cool completely before cutting.

Granola

Marge Granola, a small company based in Seattle, makes some of my favorite granola, but unfortunately, it's got more sodium than I'd like. Luckily, they shared their recipe on the Kitchn website. I tweaked it to make this "lo-so" granola.

There's lots of room to play in this recipe. Don't like cardamom? Switch it out for nutmeg, allspice, or mace, or just use the cinnamon. Like more fruits or nuts? Add them in. Try pumpkin seeds, flaxseed, hazelnuts, or whatever you happen to have in your pantry.

Makes: About 6 cups
TOTAL SODIUM: 522 mg
SODIUM PER CUP: About 87 mg

3 cups old-fashioned rolled oats

2 to 2½ cups unsalted, untoasted nuts and seeds

½ teaspoon light salt, divided

½ teaspoon ground cardamom

¼ teaspoon ground cinnamon

½ cup oil, such as melted coconut oil or olive oil

½ cup plus 1 tablespoon liquid sweetener, such as honey or maple syrup

¾ teaspoon vanilla extract

¾ cup chopped dried fruit

1   Preheat the oven to 350 degrees F and line a baking sheet with parchment paper.

2   In a large bowl, combine the oats and nuts/seeds. Stir in ¼ teaspoon of the salt and the cardamom and cinnamon. Pour in the oil, sweetener, and vanilla, and stir to coat.

3   Spoon the granola onto the prepared baking sheet, spreading it out as much as possible. Bake for about 20 minutes, then check for doneness: you want it to be golden brown and fragrant. Stir the granola, and if needed, bake for another 5 to 15 minutes.

4   Remove the baking sheet from the oven, and sprinkle the granola with the remaining ¼ teaspoon of salt. Stir in the dried fruit.

5   Store cooled granola in an airtight container for 7 to 10 days.

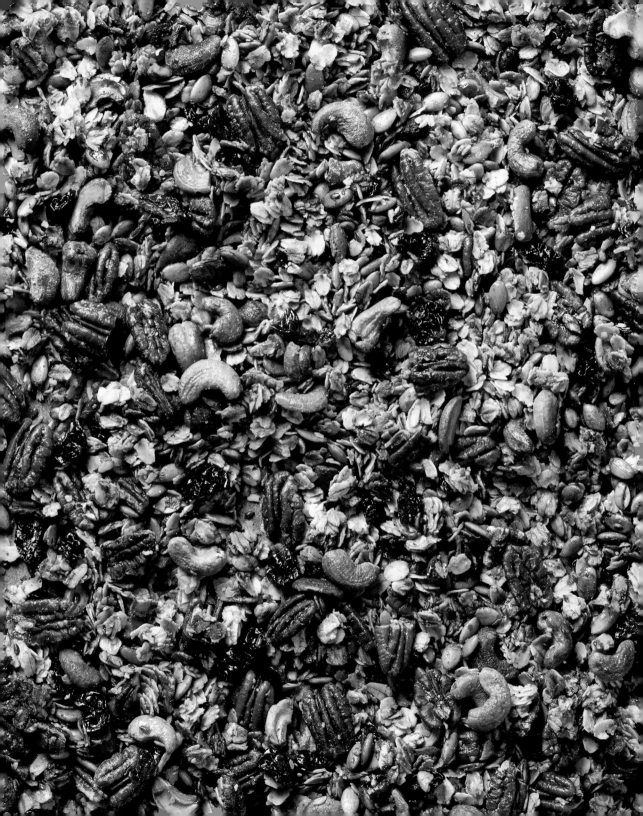

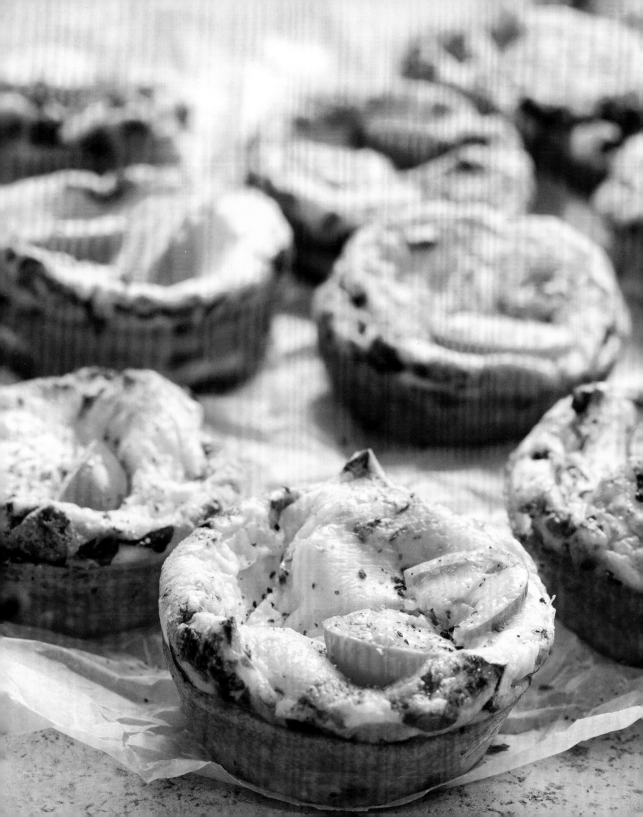

Frittata Bites

For those breakfast-on-the-go days, these frittata bites are just the thing. Just be sure not to overcook them, or they can get rubbery.

Makes: 12 mini frittatas

TOTAL SODIUM: 676 mg

SODIUM PER FRITTATA:
About 56 mg

1 tablespoon olive oil, plus more for greasing
½ cup chopped spinach

½ cup chopped cremini or button mushrooms (about 4)
¼ cup chopped onion
6 large eggs
½ cup heavy cream
6 cherry tomatoes, halved

¼ cup chopped fresh flat-leaf parsley leaves
½ teaspoon red pepper flakes
¼ teaspoon freshly ground black pepper
1 ounce freshly grated Parmesan

1   Preheat the oven to 375 degrees F and lightly grease a 12-cup muffin tin.

2   In a medium skillet, heat the oil over medium-high heat. When the oil is hot, add the spinach, mushrooms, and onion. Sauté until tender, about 5 minutes. Take the skillet off the heat and set aside.

3   In a medium bowl, whisk the eggs and cream together. Stir in the sautéed vegetables, cherry tomatoes, parsley, red pepper flakes, and black pepper.

4   Using a measuring cup to scoop the egg mixture so it doesn't splash, divide it evenly among the muffin cups. Top each cup with about ½ teaspoon of the Parmesan.

5   Bake until just set, about 10 minutes. Allow to cool for 5 minutes before serving.

6   Store in the refrigerator for up to 3 days.

Huevos Rancheros

If you are used to huevos rancheros that are more goopy cheese than eggs, you may be surprised (and hopefully, delighted) by this simpler version that skips the cheese entirely. I highly recommend using both red and green chile sauce, which I call "Christmas-style," even though I eat them that way year-round.

Makes: 1 serving

TOTAL SODIUM:
240 mg (red sauce),
229 mg (green sauce),
235 mg (half red, half green)

½ cup Red Chile Sauce (page 89) or Green Chile Sauce (page 90), or ¼ cup of each
4 tablespoons vegetable oil, divided

2 large eggs
2 corn tortillas
¼ avocado, for garnish
1 tablespoon chopped fresh cilantro leaves, for garnish

1   In a small saucepan over low heat, warm the chile sauce while you cook the eggs and tortillas.

2   In a small skillet, heat 2 tablespoons of the oil. When the oil is hot, fry the eggs to your preferred doneness. If, like me, you like yours sunny-side up, fry them for about 3 minutes.

3   In a second small skillet, heat the remaining 2 tablespoons of oil. When the oil is hot, add one of the tortillas, and fry on both sides until crisp, about 1 minute for each side. Repeat with the other tortilla.

4   To serve, place the tortillas on a plate, slightly offset. Top each tortilla with an egg, and pour the chile sauce over the top. Garnish with the avocado and cilantro.

Hash Browns

What's more tempting than a big plateful of crispy golden hash browns? Getting the flip perfected to keep the hash browns in once piece can take some practice. If you aren't confident in your flipping technique, slide the hash browns onto a plate first, then place the skillet upside down on top of the plate. With your hand on the bottom of the plate, flip the whole thing. A nonstick pan makes flipping much easier—but most nonstick pans don't brown as well.

If the whole flipping thing is just too much hassle, or if you just want individual-serving-size hash browns, fry them in smaller "pancakes" that can be flipped with a spatula.

Makes: About 2 servings

TOTAL SODIUM: 38 mg

SODIUM PER SERVING:
About 19 mg

2 medium russet
potatoes

1 medium onion
1 tablespoon safflower oil
1 tablespoon unsalted
butter

Freshly ground black
pepper
½ teaspoon red pepper
flakes

1   Using the grater disc on a food processor or the largest holes on a box grater, grate the potato and onion. Mix well. Transfer the mixture to a kitchen towel and squeeze to remove as much water as possible.

2   Line a large microwave-safe bowl with paper towels. Put the mixture in the bowl and microwave for 2 minutes.

3   In a large skillet over medium-high heat, heat the oil and butter. When the oil is hot, add the potato-onion mixture, spreading it out to evenly cover the pan. Season with the black pepper and red pepper flakes. Use a spatula to flatten. Cook until the bottom is golden, about 5 minutes, then flip.

4   Cook on the other side for another 5 minutes and serve immediately, or keep warm in a 300-degree-F oven until you are ready to serve.

Lighter Fare

Farro Salad

I like this as a hearty one-bowl lunch, but it's also great as a side dish. The nutty chew of the farro, earthy sweetness of the sweet potato, brightness of the fresh herbs, and the crunch of the nuts each contribute a panoply of flavors and textures.

You can use the farro of your choice. Here I use semi-pearled, which cooks to tenderness in about thirty minutes. Depending on your farro type, start checking for doneness after about twenty minutes.

Makes: 4 servings

TOTAL SODIUM: 205 mg

SODIUM PER SERVING: About 51 mg

1 cup farro

1 medium sweet potato, peeled and chopped into bite-size pieces

¼ cup olive oil, divided

¼ cup balsamic vinegar

1 tablespoon Mustard (page 4)

1½ cups corn kernels

1 large shallot, thinly sliced

2 tablespoons chopped fresh flat-leaf parsley leaves

2 tablespoons chopped fresh cilantro leaves

1 cup arugula

¼ cup chopped unsalted toasted nuts, such as pecans, pistachios, or almonds

2 tablespoons Chèvre (page 107)

1   Preheat the oven to 425 degrees F and line a baking sheet with parchment paper.

2   In a medium saucepan over high heat, bring 3 cups of water to a boil. Add the farro and reduce the heat to low. Simmer, uncovered, until the farro is tender, about 30 minutes. Rinse in cold water, and drain the farro well in a colander.

3   While the farro is cooking, put the sweet potato on the baking sheet. Drizzle with 1 tablespoon of the oil. Bake for 10 minutes, then stir the sweet potato. Bake for another 10 minutes, remove from the oven, and set aside to cool slightly.

4   In a small bowl, whisk together the remaining 3 tablespoons oil with the vinegar and mustard.

5   In a medium bowl, combine the farro, sweet potato, vinegar mixture, corn, shallot, parsley, and cilantro. Add the arugula, nuts, and chèvre, and gently fold to incorporate. Serve warm or at room temperature.

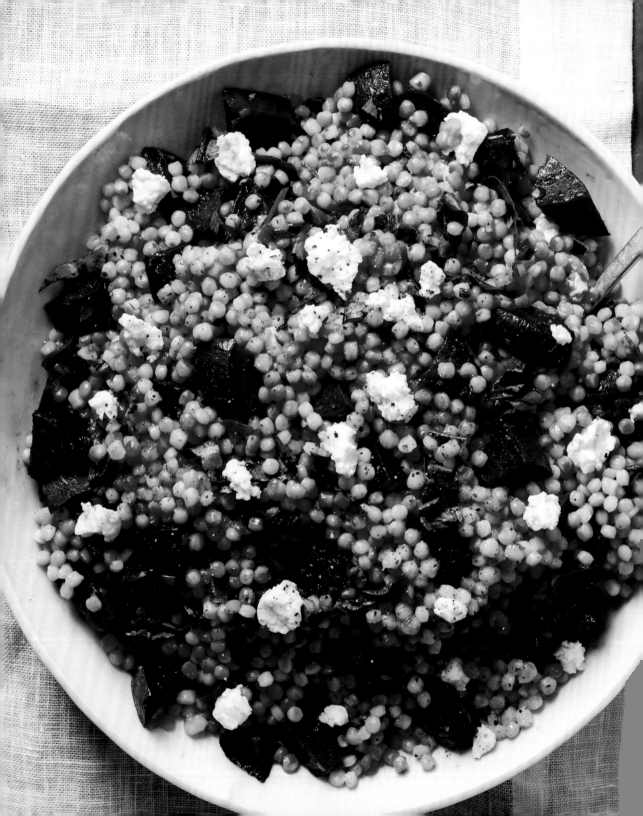

Beet & Israeli Couscous Salad

I typically prefer golden beets, but for this recipe, I use red beets because they turn the couscous a truly festive pink. If your beets don't have the greens still attached, you can toss in some arugula.

Makes: **6 servings**

TOTAL SODIUM: 419 mg

SODIUM PER SERVING:
About 70 mg

1 pound beets, with their greens
¼ cup olive oil, divided

1 tablespoon fresh thyme leaves
2 cups Israeli couscous
3 cups of water
2 tablespoons white wine vinegar
Juice of 1 medium lemon

1 cup chopped fresh flat-leaf parsley leaves
¼ cup chopped fresh chives or green onions
3 tablespoons Chèvre (page 107; optional)
Freshly ground black pepper

1   Line a baking sheet with parchment paper. Cut the beet greens from the beets and wash and drain them well. Chop them, and set aside.

2   Scrub the beets, trim away any tough parts with a knife, and chop them into bite-size pieces (no need to peel). Put them in a bowl and toss with 1 tablespoon of the oil and the thyme. Place the beets on the baking sheet in a cold oven and set the temperature to 400 degrees F. Roast until the pieces are easily pierced with a fork, 15 to 25 minutes. Remove from the oven and allow to cool.

3   Meanwhile, in a medium saucepan over medium heat, heat 1 tablespoon of the oil. When the oil is hot, add the couscous. Stir and cook until the couscous starts to become golden brown in spots, about 4 minutes. Add the water, stir, and bring to a boil. Reduce the heat to medium-low and simmer, uncovered, until the water has almost completely evaporated, about 15 minutes.

4   Rinse the couscous in cold water and drain well in a colander. Transfer the couscous to a serving bowl. Stir in the remaining 2 tablespoons oil, along with the vinegar and juice.

5   Add the beets to the couscous, along with the beet greens, parsley, chives, and chèvre. Season to taste with pepper. Serve immediately.

Vegetable Chopped Salad

This chopped salad goes low sodium by leaving out the traditional cured meat, although you could add some chopped Roasted Turkey Lunch Meat (page 103) or hard-boiled eggs if you want additional protein. For a little more zing, try marinating the chickpeas overnight in a tablespoon each of white wine vinegar and olive oil.

Makes: 2 servings

TOTAL SODIUM: 163 mg

SODIUM PER SERVING: About 81 mg

¼ cup chopped red onion

1 small head romaine or other lettuce, cored and chopped

1 avocado, diced

10 cherry tomatoes, halved

½ cup chopped cucumber

¼ cup chopped red or yellow bell pepper

2 ounces Swiss cheese, cubed (optional)

½ cup cooked Chickpeas (page 82)

¼ cup chopped fresh flat-leaf parsley leaves

¼ cup chopped fresh dill

¼ cup Balsamic Vinaigrette (page 20)

Freshly ground black pepper

¼ cup unsalted roasted pepitas, sunflower seeds, or other seeds or nuts, for garnish

1   In a small bowl, soak the onion in ice water for 5 minutes. Drain in a colander.

2   In a large bowl, toss the onion, lettuce, avocado, tomatoes, cucumber, bell pepper, Swiss cheese, chickpeas, parsley, and dill. Drizzle on the balsamic dressing and toss to coat. Season to taste with pepper and garnish with the pepitas.

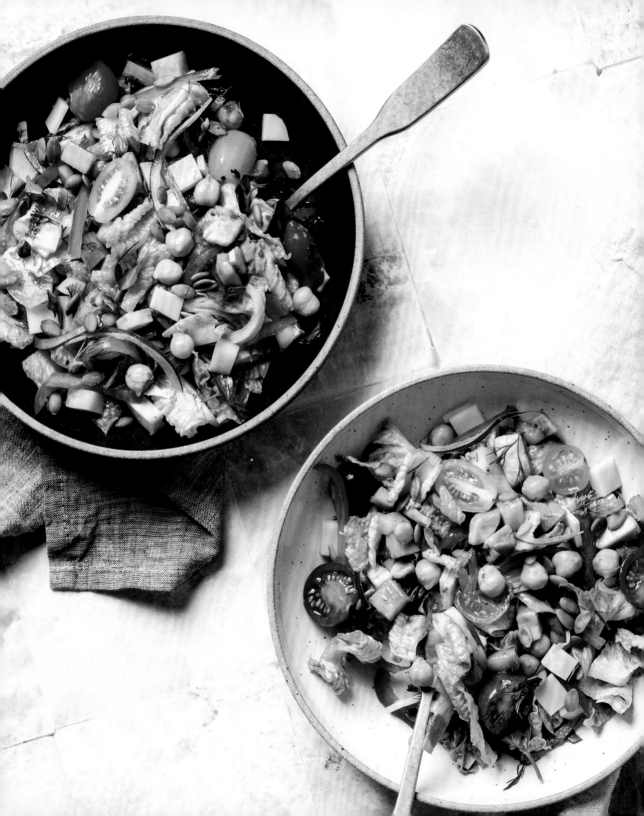

Mushroom Barley Soup

I typically use Beef Stock (page 78) made with roasted soup bones in this hearty soup, but it's equally good, though a little lighter, if you make it with Chicken Stock (page 77) or Vegetable Broth (page 79). If you use hulled barley instead of pearl barley, you will need to cook it at least thirty minutes longer on the stovetop.

Makes: About 8 cups

TOTAL SODIUM: 869 mg (beef stock), 960 mg (chicken stock), 224 mg (vegetable broth)

SODIUM PER CUP: About 109 mg (beef stock), 120 mg (chicken stock), 28 mg (vegetable broth)

1 tablespoon olive oil
1 cup pearl barley
1 cup diced onion
1 stalk celery, diced
½ pound cremini or button mushrooms, sliced
½ cup diced carrot (about 1 medium)

2 cloves garlic, minced
4 fresh sage leaves, finely chopped
1 tablespoon fresh thyme leaves
½ teaspoon freshly ground black pepper
8 cups low-sodium stock of choice

1   If you are using a multicooker, put all the ingredients in the pot. Cover, being sure to set the steam vent to closed. Cook on high pressure for 20 minutes, then let the stock naturally release according to your manufacturer's instructions, leaving the steam vent closed.

2   If you are cooking the soup on the stovetop, in a medium, heavy-bottomed soup pot over medium heat, combine the oil, barley, onion, celery, mushrooms, carrot, garlic, sage, thyme, and pepper. Sauté until the vegetables soften slightly, about 5 minutes. Add the stock, increase the heat to medium-high, and bring to a boil. Reduce the heat to medium and simmer, uncovered, for at least 30 minutes, until the barley is tender.

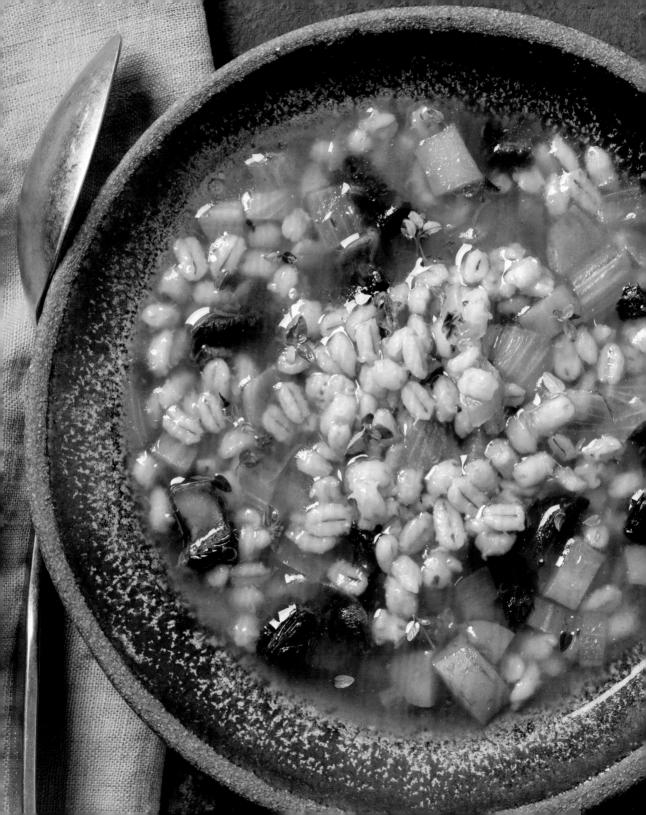

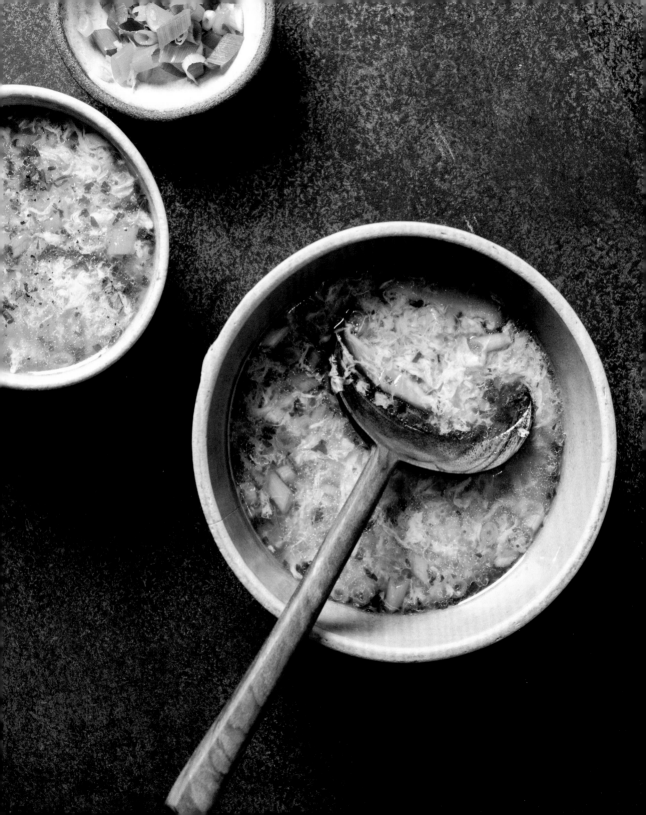

Egg Drop Soup

This version of egg drop soup is simple, but you could add tofu or corn kernels along with the mushrooms to give it more substance. Or transform it into hot-and-sour soup by adding some Sriracha (page 7) and unseasoned rice vinegar. You may be tempted to skip the cornstarch in this recipe, but that's what gives the soup its famous velvety thickness.

Makes: About 4 cups

TOTAL SODIUM: 590 mg

SODIUM PER CUP: About 147 mg

___

4 cups Chicken Stock (page 77)

1 clove garlic, minced

¾ cup sliced mushrooms

¼ cup chopped fresh cilantro leaves

1 tablespoon minced fresh ginger

1 tablespoon plus 1 teaspoon cornstarch, divided

1 tablespoon water

½ teaspoon toasted sesame oil

2 large eggs

4 green onions (light-green parts only), sliced

Freshly ground black pepper

1   In a medium soup pot over medium-high heat, combine the stock, garlic, mushrooms, cilantro, and ginger. Bring to a boil, then reduce the heat to medium and simmer for 10 minutes.

2   In a small bowl, whisk together 1 tablespoon of the cornstarch and the water. Stir it into the broth and reduce the heat to medium-low. Stir in the sesame oil.

3   In another small bowl, beat the eggs with the remaining teaspoon of cornstarch. Gradually pour the mixture into the soup, stirring slowly with chopsticks until the eggs resemble ribbons. Stir in the green onions and season to taste with pepper. Serve immediately.

Green Gazpacho

This is a low-sodium twist on my green gazpacho recipe from *An Avocado a Day*. Rice vinegar, a bit more lime juice, and a handful of Thai basil or mint make for a delightfully refreshing and zesty bowlful that I just can't get enough of. It's perfect for hot summer days.

Makes: About 5 cups
TOTAL SODIUM: 367 mg
SODIUM PER CUP: About 73 mg

3 cups diced honeydew melon (from about ½ melon)
3 tablespoons freshly squeezed lime juice
2 tablespoons freshly squeezed lemon juice
2 tablespoons unseasoned rice vinegar
2 tablespoons olive oil
1 jalapeño, seeded and chopped
1 clove garlic, minced
½ cup fresh Thai basil or mint leaves, plus more for garnish
1 avocado, diced
1 cup peeled and diced cucumber (about 1 medium)
¼ cup diced red onion
¼ teaspoon light salt
Freshly ground black pepper

1   In a blender, puree the honeydew, lime and lemon juices, vinegar, oil, jalapeño, garlic, and basil until smooth.

2   Pour the soup into a large bowl, and stir in the avocado, cucumber, onion, and salt. Season to taste with pepper. Cover the bowl with plastic wrap, pushing the wrap onto the surface of the soup to prevent it from oxidizing. Refrigerate for at least 1 hour or up to 12 hours before serving. Garnish with the basil leaves.

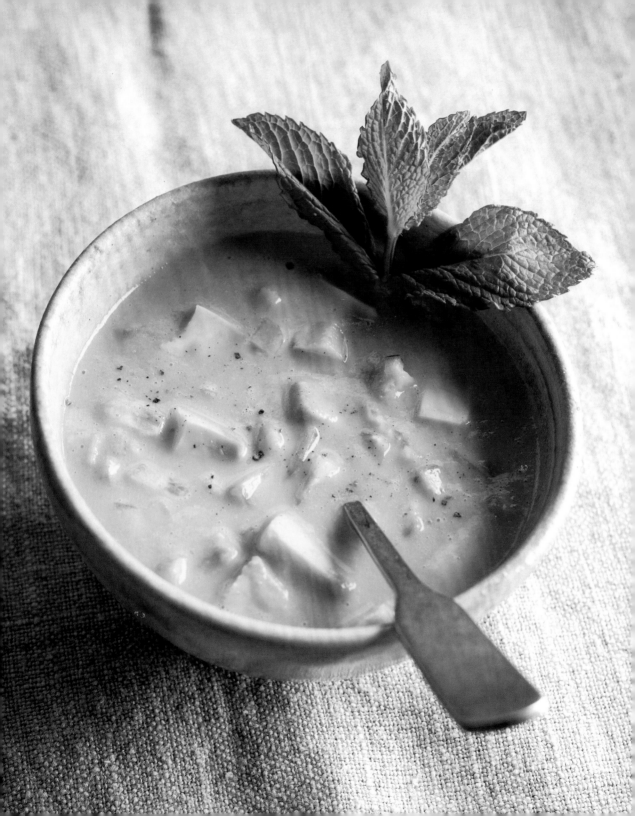

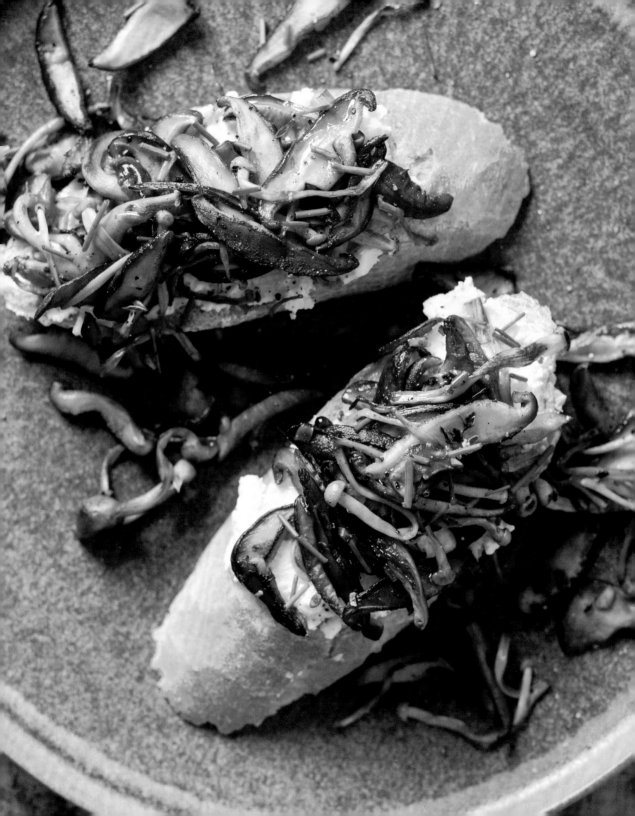

Seared Mushroom Toast

You can use just about any fresh mushroom for this toast, but it's fun to mix it up with a combination of shiitakes, maitakes, and enokis. Just slice mushrooms that are cremini size or larger. If you can get your hands on black (fermented) garlic, use it instead of the fresh garlic. It will add a lovely savory-sweet richness.

Makes: 1 serving

TOTAL SODIUM: 195 mg

1 tablespoon unsalted butter

4 ounces fresh mushrooms

1 clove garlic, minced

1 teaspoon fresh thyme leaves

Freshly ground black pepper

1 tablespoon balsamic vinegar

2 ounces Chèvre (page 107)

1 (4-inch) piece Baguette, halved lengthwise (page 49)

1 tablespoon chopped fresh chives, for garnish

1 tablespoon olive oil, for garnish

1 In a medium skillet over medium heat, melt the butter. Add the mushrooms and increase the heat to medium-high. Cook until the mushrooms are golden brown all over, stirring occasionally, about 5 minutes. Add the garlic and thyme, season to taste with pepper, and sauté until fragrant, about 1 minute. Add the vinegar and cook, stirring occasionally, until it is absorbed.

2 Spread each baguette slice with half the chèvre and top with the mushrooms. Garnish with the chives and olive oil.

Club Sandwich

Low-sodium bacon really shines in this sandwich. It provides just the right smoky crispness, and there are enough other flavors going on that you won't miss the saltiness of regular bacon.

If you aren't making your own low-sodium turkey meat, be sure to ask about low-sodium turkey at the supermarket deli counter. I haven't found many low-sodium options in the packaged lunch meat section.

Makes: **1 sandwich**

TOTAL SODIUM: 225 mg

3 slices Honey Whole Wheat Sandwich Bread (page 43)

2 tablespoons Mayonnaise (page 5)

2 leaves romaine or other large-leaf lettuce

2 slices tomato

2 pieces Bacon (page 98), halved

2 ounces sliced Roasted Turkey Lunch Meat (page 103)

1   Toast the bread and spread the mayonnaise equally over each slice.

2   Place a lettuce leaf on one of the slices of toast, followed by a slice of tomato, half of the bacon, and two slices of the turkey. Top with one of the toast slices, mayo side up. Top with the remaining lettuce, tomato, bacon, and turkey, followed by the final slice of toast, mayo side down. Gently press down on the sandwich. If you have them, use toothpicks to help secure the sandwich, and cut it into halves or quarters.

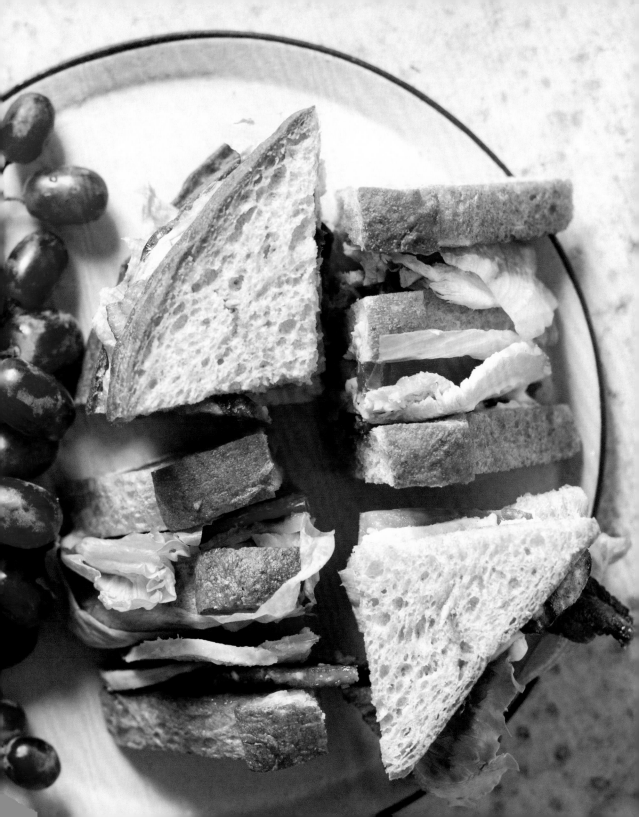

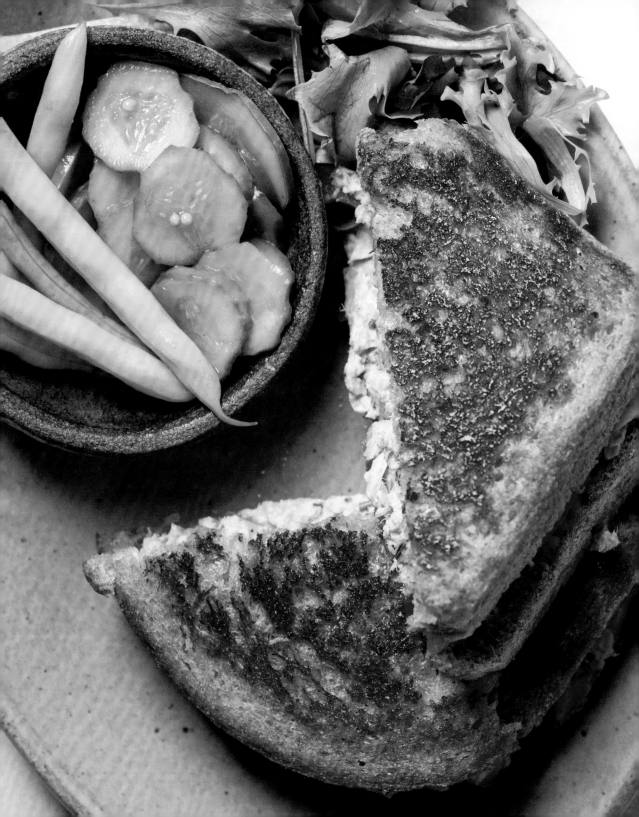

Tuna Melt

If you thought you could never have a tuna melt again, I have good news for you. Swiss cheese (and low-sodium bread and mayo) saves the day! This sandwich is comfort-food perfection. Don't like tuna? Leave out the tuna salad, slap on another slice or two of Swiss, and you've got a great grilled tomato and cheese sandwich.

Makes: 1 sandwich
TOTAL SODIUM: 225 mg

1 (2½-ounce) can unsalted albacore tuna in water, drained
1 tablespoon Mayonnaise (page 5)
1 tablespoon minced shallot
1 tablespoon freshly squeezed lemon juice
1 teaspoon balsamic vinegar
1 teaspoon Mustard (page 4)
1 teaspoon chopped fresh flat-leaf parsley leaves
1 tablespoon unsalted butter
2 slices Honey Whole Wheat Sandwich Bread (page 43)
1 slice tomato
1 slice Swiss cheese

1   In a small bowl, mix the tuna, mayonnaise, shallot, juice, vinegar, mustard, and parsley.

2   Butter one side of each slice of bread, and place one of the slices butter side down in a small skillet. Top with the tuna mixture, the tomato, and the cheese. Top with the remaining slice of bread, butter side up.

3   Put the skillet on the stove over medium-low heat and cook until the sandwich is golden brown on the bottom, about 2 minutes. Using a spatula, flip the sandwich and cook until the cheese has melted and the bottom is golden brown, about another 2 minutes. Slice in half to serve.

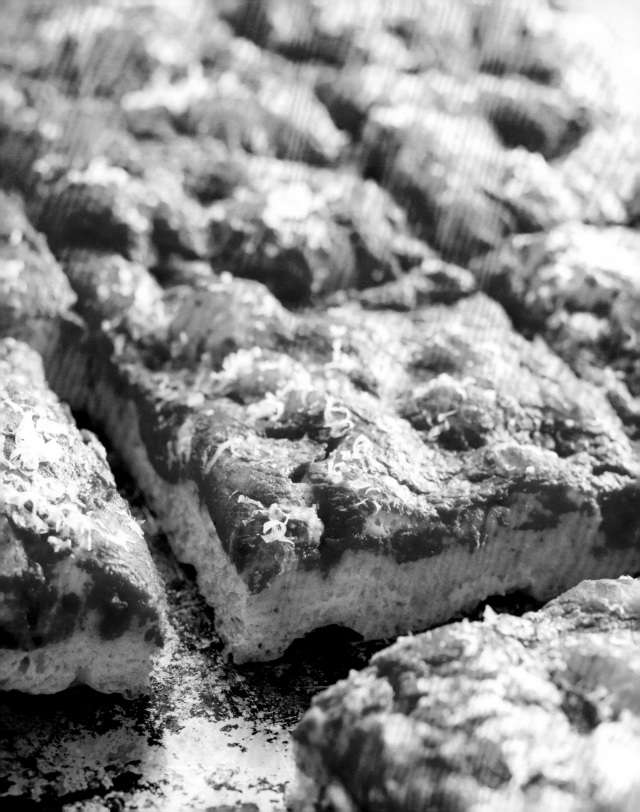

Tomato Pie

We call this "cold square pizza" in our house, but it's probably more widely known as tomato pie (a.k.a. Italian tomato pie or Philadelphia tomato pie). My husband, Cameron, first introduced me to this treat at Roma Bakery & Deli in Hamilton, Ontario, and I was immediately hooked. Luckily, it's pretty easy to make low sodium and it will sate most of your pizza cravings.

Makes: One 11-by-17-inch pie (about 12 slices)

TOTAL SODIUM: 398 mg
SODIUM PER SLICE: About 33 mg

---

3 tablespoons olive oil, divided

1 batch Focaccia dough (page 56), prepared up to the point of the first rest
1¼ cups tomato puree
3 tablespoons tomato paste
1 teaspoon red wine vinegar

1 teaspoon granulated sugar
½ ounce grated Parmesan cheese (optional)
Pinch of red pepper flakes (optional)

1 Grease an 11-by-17-inch rimmed baking sheet with 2 tablespoons of the oil.

2 Turn the dough out onto a lightly floured surface. Form it a ball, flatten the ball with your palm, and transfer it to the baking sheet. Using your hands, coat the ball on all sides with the remaining tablespoon of oil. Loosely cover the baking sheet with plastic wrap and let the dough rise in a warm place for 1 hour.

3 When the dough has risen, uncover it and, using your fingertips, press indentations across the entire surface, spreading the dough out over the baking sheet. Lightly cover, and let it rise again in a warm place for 30 minutes.

4 While the dough is on its second rise, preheat the oven to 450 degrees F.

continued

5   In a small saucepan over medium heat, combine the tomato puree, tomato paste, vinegar, and sugar. Simmer until the sugar has dissolved, about 1 minute. Set aside.

6   When the dough has risen a second time, use your fingertips to gently press indentations over the surface again. Using a spoon, spread the sauce evenly over the top of the dough, leaving a ¼-inch border. Bake until the crust is golden brown on the edges, 18 to 20 minutes.

7   Remove from the oven and sprinkle the cheese and red pepper flakes over the top. Let the pie cool to room temperature before slicing and serving.

Sriracha Chicken Wings

Need to bring a dish to your Sportball party, and want it to be something that both you and your sodium-loving friends can enjoy? These spicy wings should do the trick.

You'll only use the larger two portions of the chicken wings for this recipe, so if you are buying them whole, cut each wing into three sections at the joints and keep just the drumette and wingette.

Makes: 24 wing pieces
TOTAL SODIUM: 872 mg
SODIUM PER WING PIECE:
About 36 mg

---

24 chicken wing pieces
1 tablespoon vegetable
 oil, for greasing

⅓ cup Sriracha (page 7)
1 tablespoon unseasoned
 rice vinegar
1 tablespoon freshly
 squeezed lime juice
1 tablespoon honey

1 clove garlic, minced
2 tablespoons unsalted
 butter
½ tablespoon sesame
 seeds, for garnish

1   Preheat the oven to 500 degrees F.

2   Line a baking sheet with aluminum foil, and lightly grease the foil with the oil. Place the wings on the baking sheet, leaving about 1 inch between the pieces. Let them sit for a few minutes to lightly dry.

3   Bake, checking every few minutes, until the wings are well browned, about 10 minutes total. Using tongs, flip the wings, and bake, checking frequently, until well browned, about another 10 minutes.

4   In a small saucepan over medium heat, combine the Sriracha, vinegar, lime juice, honey, and garlic. Add the butter and continue to stir until the butter has melted. Transfer about half the sauce to a large bowl.

5   Add the wings to the bowl with the sauce and, using a spoon, turn them to coat with the sauce. Set the oven to broil, put the wings back on the baking sheet, and broil until sizzling, 2 to 3 more minutes. Watch carefully so they don't burn.

6   Sprinkle with the sesame seeds, and serve immediately, with the remaining sauce on the side.

Beans & Rice

This vegetarian dish takes its cue from Creole red beans and rice, but omits the traditional tasso ham to help bring down the sodium count. It's great as a side or even a main; you can also pile on toppings such as avocado slices, mixed spring greens, sliced cherry tomatoes, and cooked sweet potato to make a hearty grain bowl.

You won't be sorry if you seek out Carolina Gold rice, which is nuttier than many long-grain rice varieties. And give it a try with other beans, such as black or great northern beans.

Makes: 6 servings

TOTAL SODIUM: 111 mg (vegetable broth), 282 mg (chicken stock)

SODIUM PER SERVING: About 18 mg (vegetable broth), 47 mg (chicken stock)

---

1 tablespoon olive oil
1 red bell pepper, chopped
1 medium onion, chopped
3 cloves garlic, chopped
1 cup uncooked Carolina Gold or other long-grain rice
2 cups Vegetable Broth (page 79) or Chicken Stock (page 77)
½ cup water
2 tablespoons Cajun Seasoning (page 37)
2 tablespoons tomato paste
2 cups cooked kidney beans (see page 80) or Black Beans (page 86)
½ cup chopped fresh cilantro leaves
Freshly ground black pepper

1   In a large, heavy-bottomed skillet, heat the oil over medium-low heat. When the oil is hot, add the bell pepper and onion and sauté until softened, about 5 minutes. Add the garlic and rice and continue to sauté until the rice is slightly browned, another 5 minutes. Stir in the broth, water, Cajun seasoning, and tomato paste. Increase the heat to medium-high and bring to a simmer. Simmer for 5 minutes, then stir in the beans. Reduce the heat to low, cover the skillet, and simmer until the rice is cooked, about 20 minutes.

2   Use a fork to fluff the rice, and stir in the cilantro. Season to taste with pepper. Serve immediately.

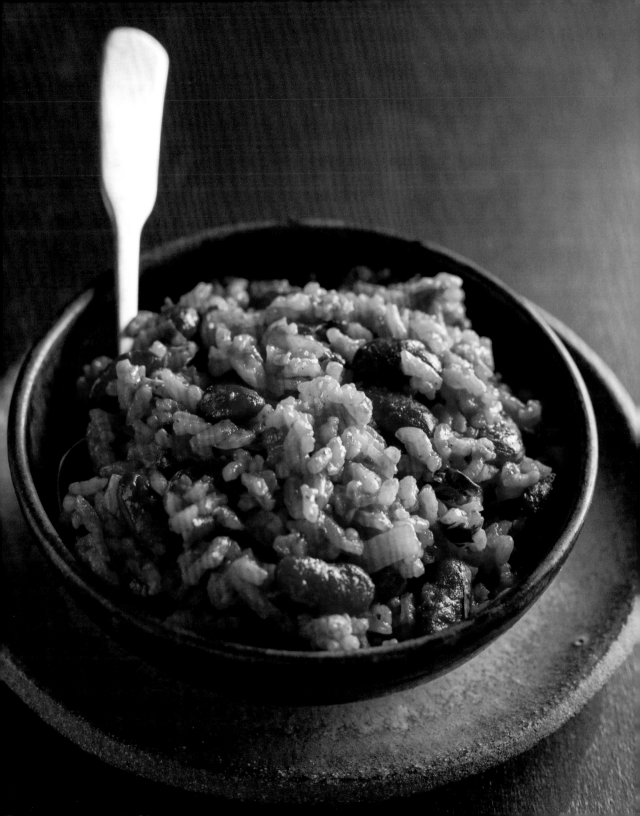

Mains

Chicken & Rice Stew

Making Chicken Stock (page 77) always results in lots of leftover bits of meat, which are perfect for this hearty stew. It's my version of chicken noodle soup.

The stew thickens when refrigerated, so if you are eating it on day two, add a bit of water when you reheat it to loosen it up, or eat it as more of a rice pilaf.

Makes: 2 large bowls
TOTAL SODIUM: 407 mg
SODIUM PER SERVING:
About 204 mg

1 teaspoon olive oil
¼ cup finely chopped onion

1 stalk celery, finely chopped
½ cup uncooked long-grain rice
¼ cup dry sherry or dry white wine
3 cups Chicken Stock (page 77)

½ cup shredded low-sodium chicken
¼ cup chopped fresh flat-leaf parsley leaves
Pinch of sumac
Freshly ground black pepper

1   In a small, heavy-bottomed saucepan, heat the oil over medium heat. When the oil is hot, add the onion and celery, and cook, stirring occasionally, until the vegetables soften, about 5 minutes. Add the rice, and cook until it is lightly toasted, 2 minutes. Add the sherry and stir to loosen any browned bits from the bottom of the pot. Add 2 cups of the chicken stock and bring to a boil over high heat, then reduce the heat to medium-high and simmer, uncovered, until the rice expands and softens, about 10 minutes. Add the chicken and parsley, and as much of the remaining cup of chicken stock as needed to reach the desired soupiness.

2   Add the sumac and season to taste with pepper. Serve immediately.

One-Pot Chicken

This is my go-to, no-brainer, weeknight dinner. It's a low-sodium version of a Jamie Oliver recipe I found on the Food52 website. The tomatoes, garlic, and basil create a simple, light sauce without any work—just toss everything in, and it comes out like magic.

I usually make it with great northern beans or chickpeas, but any firm-skinned bean would work. Feel free to up the veggie quotient by adding in some chopped squash, eggplant, or kale along with the tomatoes. It's also great served over pasta, if you want to stretch the servings a bit further.

Makes: 4 servings

TOTAL SODIUM: 924 mg

SODIUM PER SERVING: About 231 mg

2 pounds boneless, skinless chicken thighs (6 to 8)

3 cups cooked great northern beans (see page 80) or Chickpeas (page 82), drained

1 cup cherry tomatoes, halved

4 cloves garlic, peel left on and slightly smashed

⅓ cup loosely packed basil leaves

Large pinch of red pepper flakes

Freshly ground black pepper

1 tablespoon olive oil

1   Preheat the oven to 375 degrees F.

2   Put the chicken in a large Dutch oven or other oven-safe dish. Top with the beans, tomatoes, garlic, basil, and red pepper flakes. Using a spoon, push some of the beans and tomatoes underneath the chicken. Season to taste with black pepper, and drizzle the oil over the top.

3   Bake, uncovered, until a meat thermometer inserted into a thigh registers 165 degrees F, about 30 minutes. Turn on the broiler and broil, checking frequently, until the chicken is golden, about 2 minutes. Serve immediately.

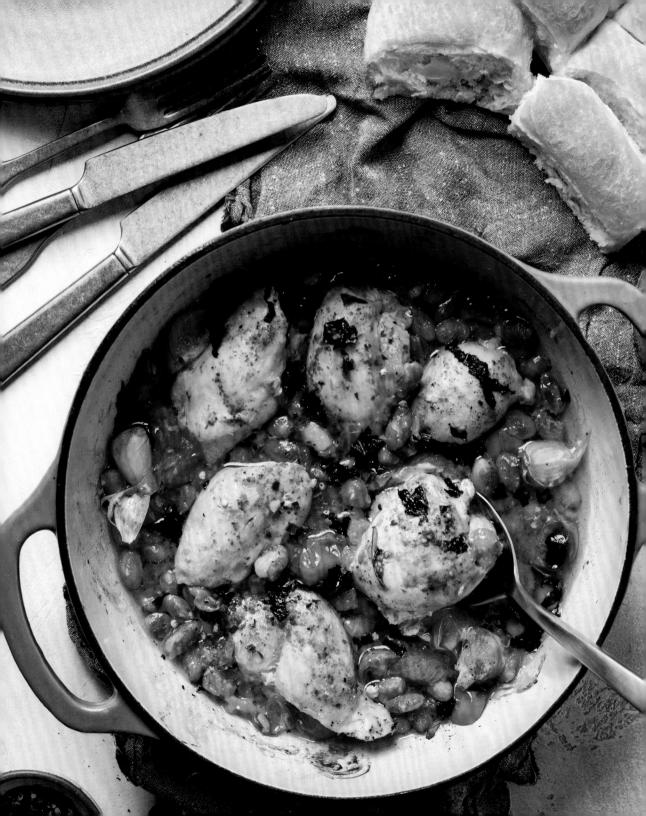

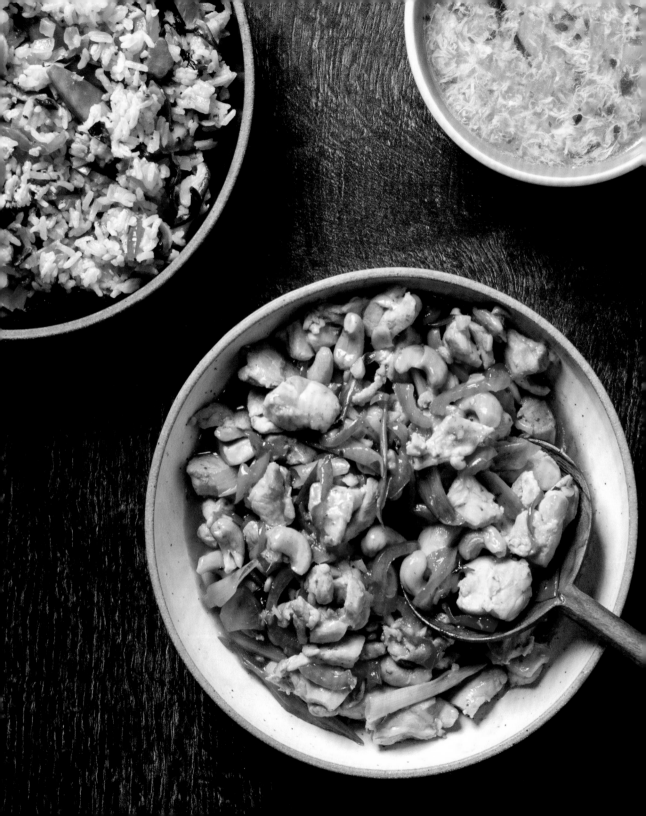

Cashew Chicken

Chinese takeout may no longer be an option for you, but that doesn't mean you can't enjoy some of the classics. Pair this easy cashew chicken with some Vegetable Fried Rice (page 221) and Egg Drop Soup (page 139).

Makes: 4 servings
TOTAL SODIUM: 820 mg
SODIUM PER SERVING:
   About 205 mg

1 bunch green onions
¾ cup Chicken Stock (page 77)
1 tablespoon coconut aminos
1 tablespoon toasted sesame oil

1½ teaspoons cornstarch
1 teaspoon granulated sugar
3 tablespoons sunflower or other vegetable oil
1 pound skinless, boneless chicken thighs or breasts, cut into ¾-inch cubes

1 red bell pepper, chopped
4 cloves garlic, finely chopped
1½ tablespoons finely chopped fresh ginger
¼ teaspoon red pepper flakes
½ cup unsalted roasted whole cashews

1   Trim the ends and any tough tops from the green onions. Chop the green onions on an angle and separate the green and white parts. Set aside.

2   In a small bowl, mix the chicken stock, coconut aminos, sesame oil, cornstarch, and sugar. Set aside.

3   In a wok over high heat, add the oil, and swirl it around the wok to coat. Add the chicken, and stir-fry until golden, 4 to 5 minutes. Use a slotted spoon to remove the chicken to a plate and set aside.

4   Add the white parts of the green onion, along with the bell pepper, garlic, ginger, and red pepper flakes, and stir-fry until fragrant, about 2 minutes. Add the chicken stock mixture and stir-fry until the liquid thickens slightly, about 2 minutes. Add the chicken back to the wok with the green parts of the green onion and the cashews, and stir-fry until the chicken is hot, another 2 to 3 minutes. Serve immediately.

Chicken Chana Masala

A multicooker, such as an Instant Pot, makes quick work of infusing flavors and tenderizing the chicken in this classic Indian curry.

Makes: 6 servings
TOTAL SODIUM: 1,256 mg
SODIUM PER SERVING:
About 209 mg

2 tablespoons ghee or olive oil
1 medium onion, diced
2 cloves garlic, minced
2 teaspoons grated fresh ginger
1½ teaspoons smoked paprika

1½ teaspoons ground coriander
1 teaspoon ground turmeric
1 teaspoon ground cumin
½ teaspoon freshly ground black pepper
¼ teaspoon cayenne pepper
2 cups tomato puree
2 cups trimmed and chopped kale or spinach

2½ pounds (about 8) boneless chicken thighs
1 cup chopped fresh cilantro leaves
2 cups cooked Chickpeas (page 82)
¼ cup freshly squeezed lemon juice (from 2 medium lemons)
¼ cup heavy cream

1   In a pressure cooker over medium-high heat (or using the Sauté function on a multicooker) or in a 4-quart pot, heat the ghee. Add the onion, garlic, and ginger, and sauté until the onion softens, about 5 minutes. Add the paprika, coriander, turmeric, cumin, black pepper, and cayenne pepper and cook until the spices are lightly toasted, about 2 minutes. Add the tomato puree and kale and cook until the kale has wilted, another 5 minutes.

2   Add the chicken and cilantro, then cover, being sure to set the steam vent to closed. Cook on high pressure for 15 minutes. Allow the pressure to release naturally and remove the lid. If cooking on the stovetop, cover and cook over medium heat for 50 minutes, or until the chicken pieces are cooked through.

3   Stir in the chickpeas, lemon juice, and heavy cream, and set the pressure cooker back over medium heat (or use the Sauté function). Cook until the sauce thickens, about 5 minutes. Serve immediately.

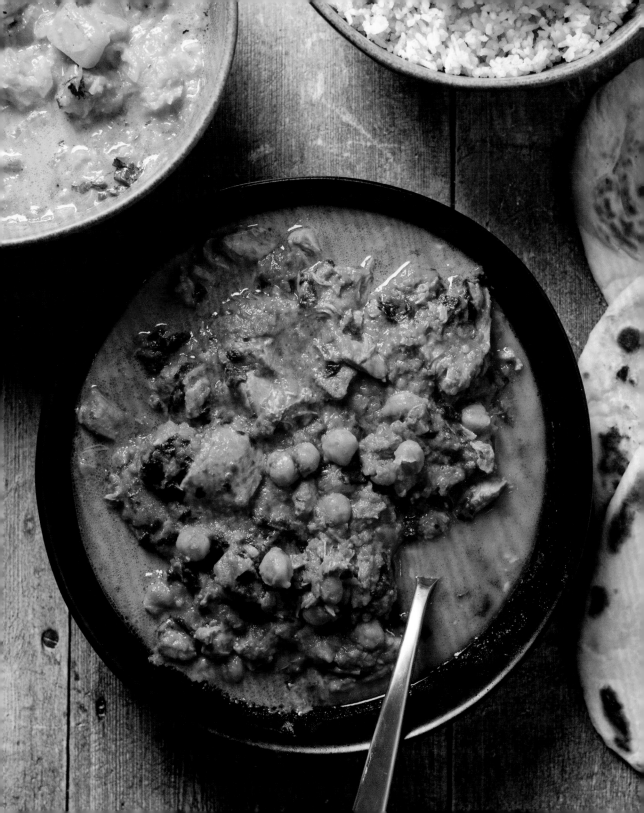

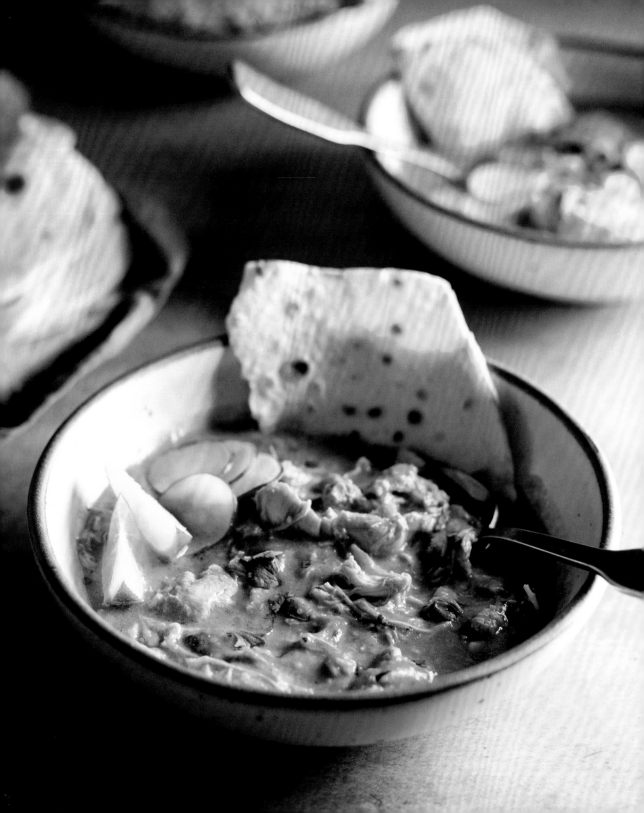

Chicken Chile Verde

I adapted this dish—quick, easy, and the perfect warm-you-up meal—from one of my favorite recipes on Serious Eats. That recipe uses fish sauce, which is pretty much a no-no for those of us on a low-sodium diet, but a tablespoon of coconut aminos makes a nice substitution. The original recipe was made with pork shoulder, and you can easily swap out the chicken thighs here with two pounds of pork shoulder, cut into 2-inch chunks.

This recipe is designed for a multicooker, but if you don't have one, you can make it in a slow cooker. Just combine all the ingredients, plus a pint of chicken stock, into the slow cooker and cook on high for about three hours.

Serve with Flour Tortillas (page 61) to sop up all the sauce.

Makes: 4 servings

TOTAL SODIUM: 1,191 mg

SODIUM PER SERVING: About 298 mg

___

1 tablespoon olive oil

2 pounds (about 6) boneless, skinless chicken thighs

2 poblano peppers, stemmed, seeded, and roughly chopped

2 Anaheim chilies, stemmed, seeded, and roughly chopped

2 jalapeños, stemmed, seeded, and roughly chopped

1 medium onion, roughly chopped

3 cloves garlic, peeled

¼ pound tomatillos, peeled and chopped (optional)

1 teaspoon ground cumin

¼ cup coarsely chopped fresh cilantro leaves

1 tablespoon coconut aminos

Freshly ground black pepper

1 medium lime, quartered, for serving

1   In a multicooker on the Sauté function (or over high heat if you are using a stove-top pressure cooker), heat the oil. When the oil is hot, add the chicken, peppers, chilies, jalapeños, onion, garlic, tomatillos, and cumin. Stir a little to mix everything up. Cover, being sure to set the steam vent to closed, and cook on high pressure for 30 minutes.

continued

2   Allow the pressure to release naturally and remove the lid. Using a slotted spoon, transfer the chicken thighs to a large bowl and set aside.

3   Add the cilantro and coconut aminos to the pot with the sauce. Use an immersion blender to puree the mixture until it is smooth. Season to taste with black pepper. Return the chicken to the sauce, and simmer for about 5 minutes. Ladle the chicken and a healthy serving of sauce into individual bowls, and serve immediately with the lime wedges.

4   You'll likely have leftover chile verde sauce. Save it and pile it on eggs, or serve it with some unsalted tortilla chips.

Chicken Potpie

While my mother made her own pies quite frequently, for some reason, potpies in our house tended to be the frozen variety. I do still have a nostalgic fondness for those, but this savory pie's crust is delightfully flaky instead of cardboard-like, and the fresh herbs and vegetables in the filling is pure comfort without the heaviness.

Because this is a top-crust-only potpie, it only uses a half recipe of pie dough, but I recommend making a full batch and freezing one of the two dough discs for later use, keeping the other refrigerated until you are ready to make the potpie.

Makes: 4 servings

TOTAL SODIUM: 934 mg

SODIUM PER SERVING: About 234 mg

½ recipe Pie Dough (page 73), chilled

3 tablespoons olive oil

1 medium onion, diced

1 medium yellow potato, diced

½ cup diced carrot (about 1 medium)

2 cloves garlic, minced

1 tablespoon chopped fresh flat-leaf parsley leaves

1 teaspoon fresh thyme leaves

1 teaspoon chopped fresh rosemary

3 tablespoons all-purpose flour

1 cup dry white wine

3 cups (1 pound) shredded unsalted chicken meat

2 cups Chicken Stock (page 77)

½ cup fresh or frozen peas

1 large egg

1 tablespoon water

1   Heat the oven to 450 degrees F and line a baking sheet with parchment paper.

2   In a large cast-iron skillet over medium heat, heat the oil. When the oil is hot, add the onion, potato, and carrot. Cook until the onion is translucent, about 10 minutes. Add the garlic, parsley, thyme, and rosemary. Cook until softened, another 10 minutes.

continued

3   Stir in the flour, and continue to cook, stirring constantly until the flour starts to lightly brown. Stir in the wine, and simmer for 10 minutes. Add the chicken, chicken stock, and peas. Simmer until the potatoes start to soften, another 15 minutes.

4   Meanwhile, on a generously floured work surface, roll the dough out into a 10-inch circle about ¼ inch thick. Wrapping the dough around your rolling pin, carefully transfer it to the skillet, placing it on top of the filling, with the pastry edges sloping up the edge of the pan. Make an egg wash: In a small bowl, using a fork, mix the egg with the water. Brush the top of the pastry with the egg wash and use a sharp knife to cut several vents in the pastry.

5   Put the skillet on the baking sheet. Bake for 10 minutes, then reduce the heat to 375 degrees F. Bake until the top is a deep golden brown, another 10 to 15 minutes. Serve immediately.

6   Refrigerate leftovers in the skillet, covered with aluminum foil, for up to 3 days. Reheat in a 350-degree oven for about 15 minutes.

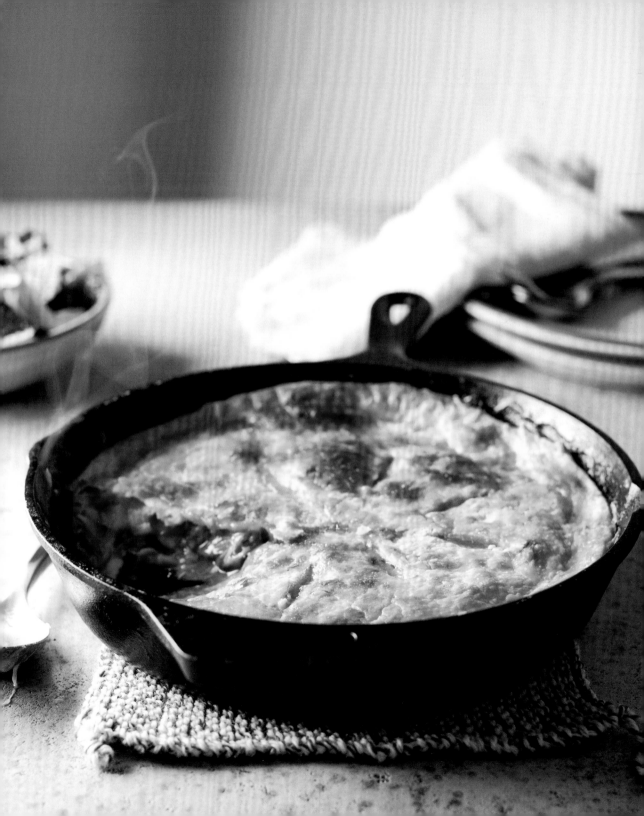

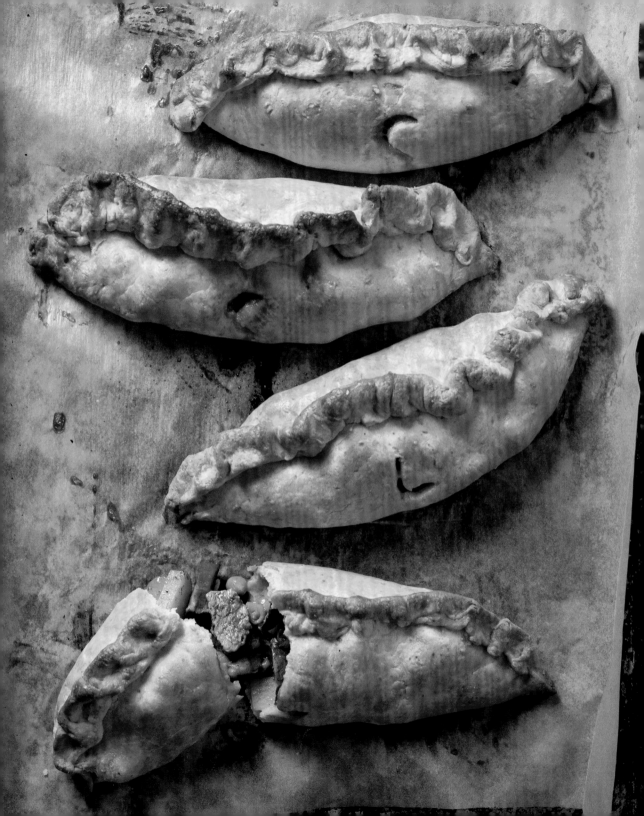

Cornish Pasties

Cornish pasties are another of the recipes from my family's repertoire. These savory pastries were traditionally eaten by miners in the copper mines of Cornwall, England, and then somehow made their way to Upper Michigan and the northern Midwest, and, along the road, to my family's table. They are similar to calzones, but packed with meat and potatoes instead of tomato and cheese. Each pastry typically has the initials of the eater carved into the top, so it's easy to customize the filling for individual tastes (for example, you could add a bit more salt to some).

Makes: 4 large pasties
TOTAL SODIUM: 431 mg
SODIUM PER PASTY: About 108 mg

FOR THE FILLING

½ pound sirloin or chuck steak, chopped into bite-size cubes
2 medium yellow potatoes, cut into ½-inch cubes
3 green onions (white and green parts), chopped
½ cup fresh or frozen peas
1 teaspoon fresh thyme leaves
Freshly ground black pepper

FOR THE PASTRY

3 cups (360 grams) all-purpose flour
½ teaspoon sodium-free baking powder
¼ teaspoon light salt
14 tablespoons unsalted butter, cold, cut into ½-inch cubes
⅔ cup ice water

1   Preheat the oven to 400 degrees F and line a baking sheet with parchment paper.

2   To make the filling, in a large bowl, mix together all the ingredients except for the pepper. Or, if you are personalizing each pasty, place each filling ingredient in a separate bowl and add to each pasty as desired. Set aside.

continued

3   To make the pastry, in another large bowl, whisk together the flour, baking powder, and salt. Use a pastry cutter to cut in the butter until the pieces are about the size of peas. Stir in the water, about 2 tablespoons at a time, until the dough comes together. You may not need all the water. Divide the dough into 4 equal balls. Cover with a towel and set aside.

4   On a lightly floured work surface, roll one of the dough balls into a circle about 6 inches wide and ¼ inch thick.

5   Add about 1 cup of filling on one side of the circle, leaving a 1-inch border. Season the filling with a twist or two of black pepper. Brush a little bit of water onto the edges of the dough. Grab the top edge of the dough, and fold it over the filling to meet the bottom edge. Crimp to seal with your fingers or a fork. With a sharp knife, cut a vent in the top of the dough (perhaps using the initials of the person eating the pasty, if personalized). Repeat with the remaining dough balls.

6   Bake until the crust is golden brown, about 1 hour. Cool for at least 15 minutes before serving.

7   Serve warm. If not serving immediately, wrap the pasties in aluminum foil; they will stay warm for more than an hour.

Italian Sausage & Mushroom Pizza

With reduced-sodium dough and sausage, and a little less cheese than usual, you can enjoy pizza again. For even more flavor, try loading it up with thinly sliced onions, fresh tomatoes, and thinly sliced peppers. (You can make it lower in sodium still by leaving out the sausage entirely.)

Be sure to use fresh mozzarella (the type that is stored in whey), which not only has considerably less sodium than its firmer counterpart, but tastes better too.

Makes: Two 12-inch pizzas
TOTAL SODIUM: 760 mg
SODIUM PER PIZZA: About 380 mg

½ recipe Pizza Dough (page 58), at room temperature

½ pound uncooked Italian Sausage (page 94)

⅓ cup low-sodium tomato sauce

3 ounces fresh mozzarella, grated

½ cup button mushrooms, thinly sliced

1 ounce grated Parmesan, for garnish

About 12 fresh basil leaves, for garnish

Red pepper flakes, for garnish

1   Divide the pizza dough into 2 pieces, and form them into balls. Cover and set aside.

2   In a medium skillet over medium heat, cook the sausage, breaking up any large pieces with a wooden spoon, until cooked through, about 5 minutes. Use a slotted spoon to remove the sausage to a plate. Set aside.

3   Preheat the oven to 550 degrees F. If you are using a pizza stone, put it in the oven while it heats. If you are using a baking sheet to bake your pizza, lightly grease it with vegetable oil, but leave it out.

continued

4   On a generously floured work surface, use your fingertips to gently flatten one of the dough balls into a circle with a bit of a ridge around the edges. Flour your hands, then pick up the dough and pass it back and forth between your palms, gently stretching and rotating the circle until it is approximately 12 inches in diameter.

5   If you are using a pizza stone, place your dough on a pizza peel, or on the back of a baking sheet dusted with cornmeal or semolina flour. Shake the peel or pan slightly to make sure the dough isn't sticking; if it is, add more cornmeal. If you are using a baking sheet, place your dough directly on the pan.

6   Spoon on half of the tomato sauce, spreading it evenly and leaving a 1-inch border around the edge. Layer on half of the mozzarella, sausage, and mushrooms.

7   To transfer the pizza to the stone, place the end of the pizza peel or baking sheet on the far edge of the stone, then pull the peel or pan toward you, letting the pizza slide onto the stone. Bake until golden brown and bubbly, about 4 minutes on a pizza stone, or 10 minutes on a baking pan. Repeat with the remaining dough ball and toppings.

8   Garnish to taste with the Parmesan, basil, and red pepper flakes, and serve immediately.

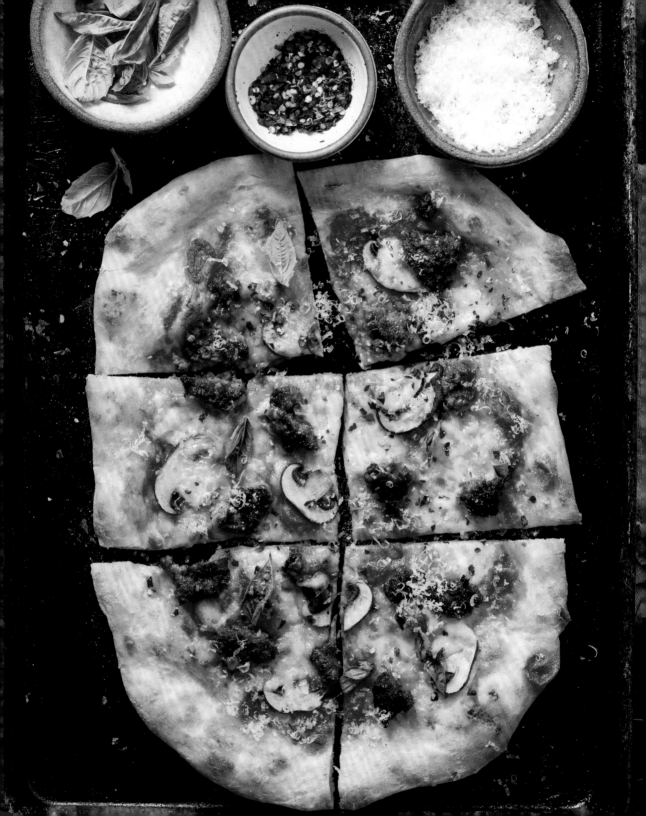

Beef & Bean Chili

This is a quick weeknight chili that is easy to throw together from things I typically have in my pantry and freezer. (It's a good reason to make a big batch of beans ahead of time and freeze them.)

If you aren't using the Taco Seasoning (page 35), be sure to check your chili powder for sodium; some contain salt. I love Rancho Gordo chili powder, which you can order from its website (and get some great beans for your chili there as well).

Brown Butter Sage Corn Bread (page 68) is the perfect accompaniment to this chili.

Makes: 4 servings

TOTAL SODIUM: 392 mg

SODIUM PER SERVING:
  98 mg

1 tablespoon olive oil
1 medium onion, diced
1 green bell pepper,
  diced

1 jalapeño, seeded and
  diced
1 clove garlic, minced
1 pound ground beef
2 cups canned unsalted
  chopped tomatoes

¼ cup Taco Seasoning
  (page 35) or salt-free
  chili powder
¼ teaspoon freshly
  ground black pepper
2 cups cooked and
  drained kidney or pinto
  beans (see page 80)

1 Heat the oil in a large skillet over medium-low heat. When the oil is hot, add the onion, bell pepper, jalapeño, and garlic. Cook, stirring frequently, until the veggies have slightly softened, about 5 minutes.

2 Increase the heat to medium-high and stir in the ground beef. Cook until the meat has browned, 5 minutes. Add the tomatoes, taco seasoning, and black pepper. Cook for about 3 minutes, then stir in the beans. Cook for another 10 minutes, adding a bit of water if needed if it gets too thick. Serve warm.

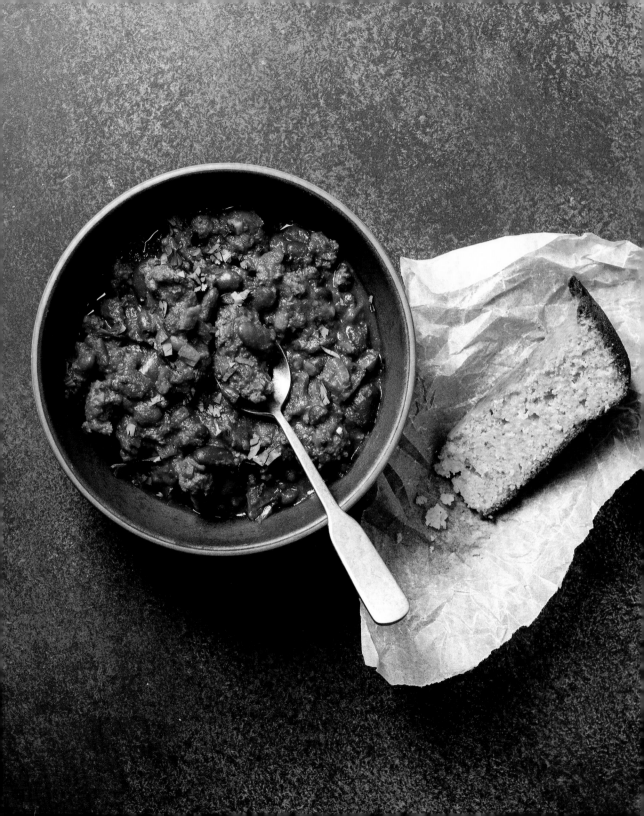

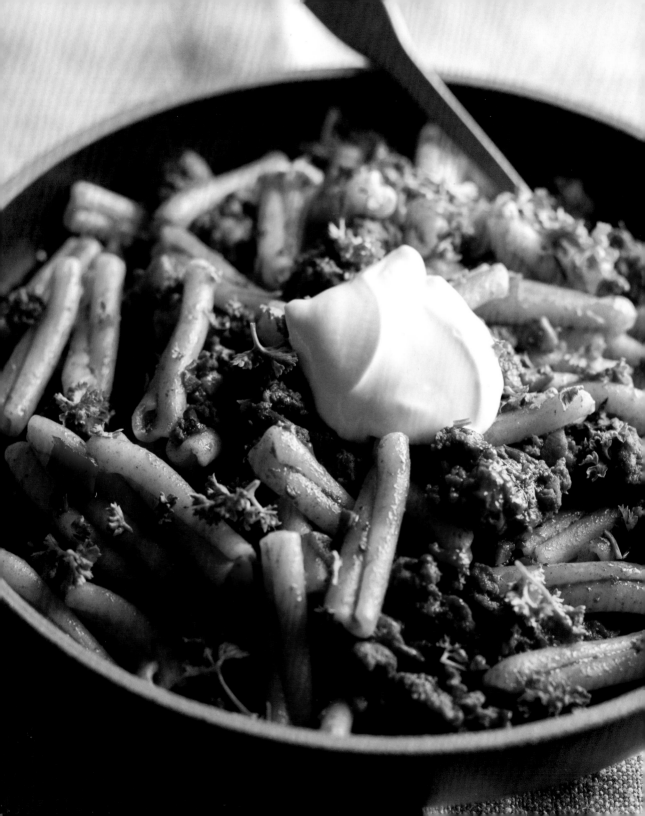

Spiced Harissa Ragù

You can make this sauce with ground beef or lamb (the sodium counts are basically the same). Lamb's stronger flavor pairs really well with the harissa, so that's usually my choice. It's one of those dishes that feels restaurant worthy, even though it's a breeze to prepare if you've made the harissa ahead of time. Don't skip the dollop of yogurt at the end: it really adds to the dish and cools the spice.

Makes: 4 servings
TOTAL SODIUM: 423 mg
SODIUM PER SERVING:
About 106 mg

2 tablespoons olive oil, divided
½ medium onion, finely chopped
1 red bell pepper, seeded and chopped
2 cloves garlic, finely chopped
8 button mushrooms, stemmed and chopped
¼ cup dry sherry
1 pound ground lamb or beef
1½ tablespoons Harissa (page 8)
½ teaspoon sumac
¼ teaspoon ground cinnamon
¼ teaspoon ground cumin
¼ teaspoon ground coriander
3 cups small-shaped pasta, such as cavatelli
½ cup yogurt
¼ cup chopped fresh flat-leaf parsley leaves
¼ cup chopped fresh cilantro leaves

1   In a small heavy pot such as a Dutch oven, heat 1 tablespoon of the oil over medium heat. When the oil is hot, add the onion and reduce the heat to medium-low. Sauté until the onion has softened, about 5 minutes. Add the bell pepper and garlic, and sauté for another 2 minutes. Add the mushrooms and increase the heat to medium-high. Cook, stirring frequently, until the mushrooms have given up most of their liquid, about 5 minutes. Stir in the sherry and scrape any brown bits off the bottom and sides of the pan.

continued

2   Add the ground lamb, breaking up any large pieces with a wooden spoon. Sauté the lamb until it is mostly browned, about 5 minutes. Stir in the harissa, sumac, cinnamon, cumin, and coriander. Continue to cook until the lamb has completely browned, about 5 minutes. Reduce the heat to low and keep the lamb mixture warm while you make the pasta.

3   In a large saucepot over high heat, bring about 6 cups of water to a boil. Add the pasta and cook until al dente according to the manufacturer's instructions, usually about 10 to 12 minutes for dried pasta.

4   Meanwhile, in a small bowl, mix the yogurt with the remaining tablespoon of oil. Set aside.

5   When the pasta is ready, drain it in a colander, reserving the pasta water. Add the pasta to the lamb mixture, stirring to coat it with the ragù. Add about ½ to 1 cup of the pasta water and cook until the water has mostly absorbed. Stir in the parsley and cilantro.

6   Serve immediately with a dollop of the yogurt sauce.

Roasted Pork Tacos

This mojo-inspired roasted pork is another great recipe for a multi-cooker: the pork ends up perfectly tender, and there is less chance of it overcooking and getting dry. A slow cooker works as well, if you want to just throw everything into a pot and have it ready to go after a few hours. You could also make this recipe as a slow braise in the oven by cooking the pork, covered with aluminum foil, for about two hours at 275 degrees F, followed by another hour, uncovered, at 325 degrees to crisp up the crust.

Makes: Enough pork for about 18 tacos

TOTAL SODIUM (PORK ONLY): 962 mg

SODIUM PER SERVING (PORK ONLY): About 53 mg

SODIUM PER TACO (WITH TORTILLAS AND TOPPINGS): About 71 mg (corn), 94 mg (flour)

2 tablespoons vegetable oil

3 pounds pork shoulder

1 medium onion, peeled and quartered

4 cloves garlic

1 dried red chili pepper, such as guajillo, stemmed and seeded

1 bay leaf

1 teaspoon coriander seeds

1 teaspoon cumin seeds

1 teaspoon smoked paprika

½ teaspoon black peppercorns

Zest and juice of 1 medium orange

Zest and juice of 1 medium lime

FOR SERVING

18 corn or Flour Tortillas (page 61)

Pico de Gallo (page 14)

Avocado slices

Lime wedges

1   In a large cast-iron pan over medium heat, heat the oil. When the oil is hot, sear the outside of the pork shoulder on all sides.

2   Transfer the pork and any fat drippings to a multicooker or slow cooker. Add the onion, garlic, chili, bay leaf, coriander and cumin seeds, paprika, peppercorns, and orange and lime zests. Lightly stir to mix everything up a bit. Pour the orange and lime juices over the top.

continued

3   If you are using a multicooker, cover, being sure to set the steam vent to closed. Cook on high pressure for 45 minutes, with a natural release. If you are using a slow cooker, cook on high for 5 hours or low for about 8 hours, or until the pork is tender. Carefully remove the pork from the cooker and roughly shred it.

4   To serve, set the oven on broil and put the shredded pork in a large casserole dish. Broil until the pork is crispy on top, about 5 minutes. Stir the pork, and broil for another 5 minutes. Warm the tortillas, fill them with pork, and serve with pico de gallo, sliced avocado, and lime wedges.

5   Leftover pork keeps well in the freezer. Allow it to cool, wrap it in plastic wrap, and freeze it for up to 2 months. Defrost in the refrigerator before using.

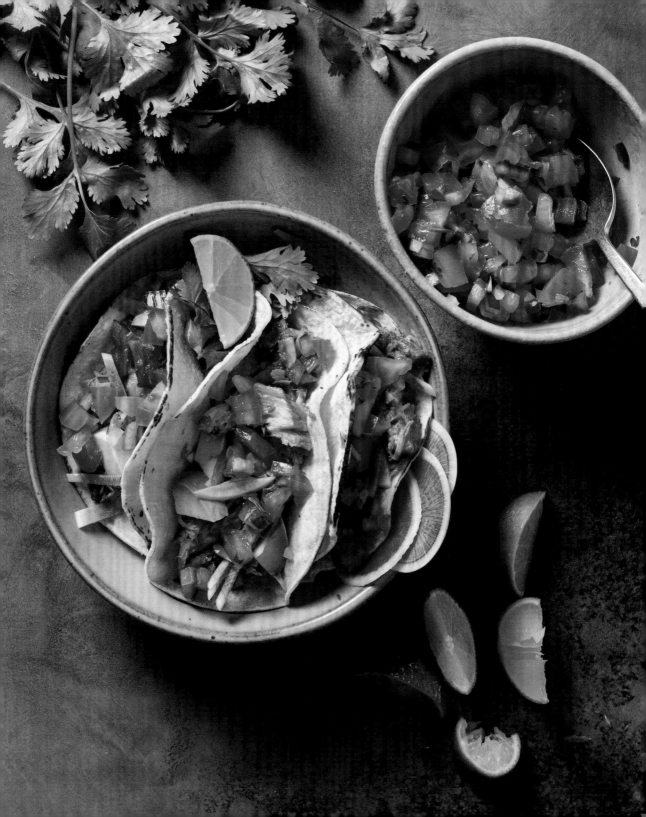

Barbecue Ribs

These ribs are fall-off-the-bone tender, thanks to the braise before they ever hit the grill. That also makes them very easy to prepare ahead of time, so they only take a few minutes over the flames.

Makes: 2 hearty servings

TOTAL SODIUM: 607 mg

SODIUM PER SERVING:
   About 303 mg

───────────

2 pounds back pork or
   beef ribs

Freshly ground black
   pepper
2 medium onions, peeled
   and quartered
2 cloves garlic
1 teaspoon dried basil

1 teaspoon dried oregano
1 teaspoon dried
   rosemary
About ⅓ cup Barbecue
   Sauce (page 9)

1   Cut the rack of ribs into strips, about 2 bones each. Season each strip with a few grinds of pepper, and put them in a large, heavy-bottomed saucepot. Cover the ribs with water and add the onions, garlic, basil, oregano, and rosemary. Over medium heat, bring to a rolling boil, then reduce the heat slightly to keep it at a low boil for an hour and a half. After 90 minutes, using tongs, carefully remove the ribs from the stock (they will be very tender at this point) to a plate.

2   If you are using a multicooker, put all the ingredients except for the barbecue sauce in the pot. Cover, being sure to set the steam vent to closed. Cook on high pressure for 25 minutes, with a natural release.

3   If you are making these ahead of time, allow the ribs to cool to room temperature before refrigerating them for up to 2 days before grilling.

4   When you are ready to grill the ribs, preheat a gas grill.

5   Cook the ribs over high heat until they brown and start to crisp, about 3 minutes on each side. Brush them with the barbecue sauce on one side and move them to a cooler section of the grill. Cook, sauced side up, on one side until the sauce starts to dry, about 2 minutes. Using tongs, turn the ribs over and brush sauce on the other side. Serve immediately.

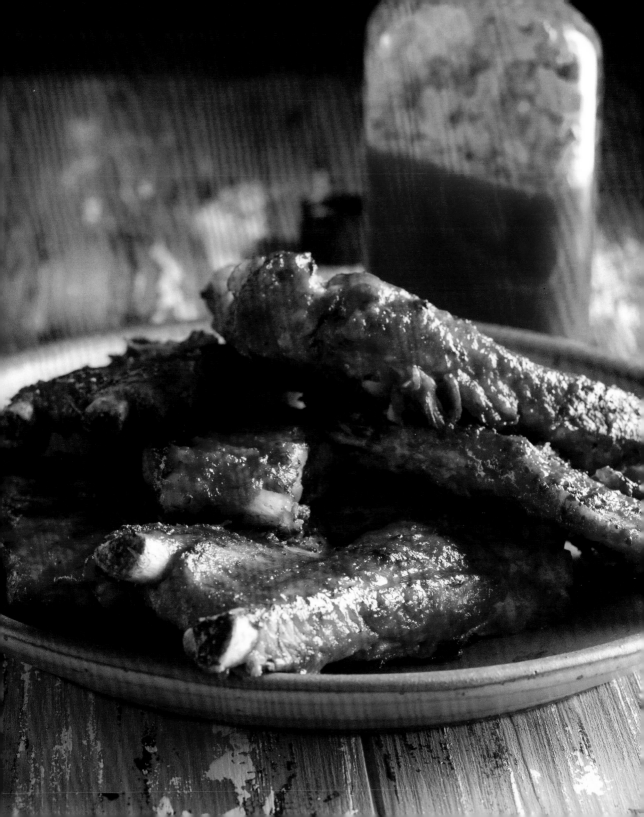

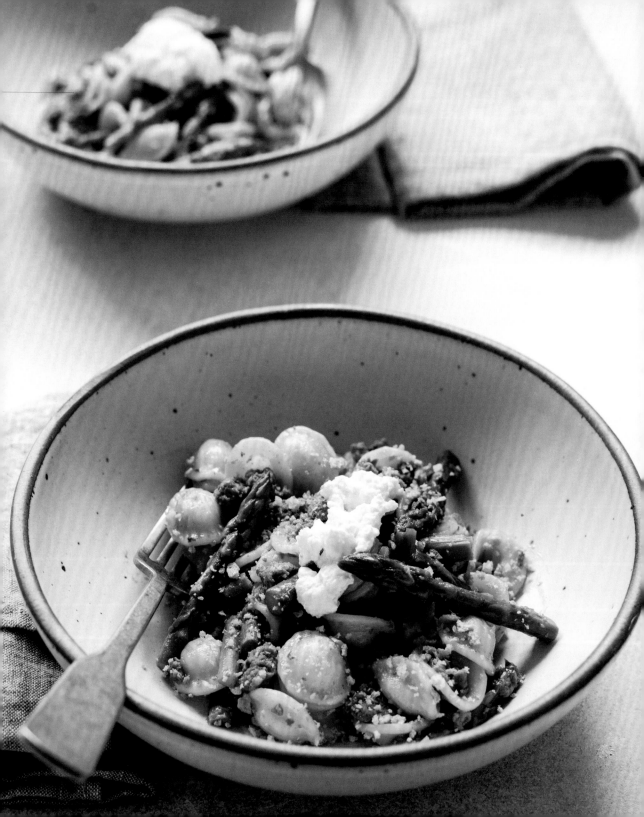

Orecchiette with Merguez & Asparagus

This pasta takes a little forethought, as you'll need to make the merguez, ricotta, and bread crumbs in advance. But with these low-sodium staples on hand, you can pull together a great meal in no time.

Makes: 2 servings
TOTAL SODIUM: 373 mg
SODIUM PER SERVING:
  About 186 mg

1 bunch asparagus, trimmed and cut into 1-inch pieces (about 1 pound)

½ pound orecchiette or other short pasta
2 tablespoons olive oil, divided
2 cloves garlic, minced
Zest and juice of 1 medium lemon

½ pound Merguez (page 101)
Freshly ground black pepper
½ cup Ricotta (page 105)
½ cup toasted bread crumbs (see page 52)

1   Fill a medium saucepot with water and bring to a boil over high heat.

2   Blanch the asparagus in the boiling water for about 1 minute, then use a slotted spoon to remove the pieces to a plate. Set aside.

3   Add the pasta to the pot and cook until al dente according to the manufacturer's instructions, usually about 10 to 12 minutes for dried pasta.

4   While the pasta cooks, in a large sauté pan, heat 1 tablespoon of the oil over medium heat. When the oil is hot, add the garlic and cook until the garlic has started to soften, about 5 minutes. Add the asparagus, and cook until it softens slightly, about 5 minutes. Stir in the lemon zest, then transfer the mixture to a bowl. Set aside.

5   Heat the remaining tablespoon of oil in the sauté pan. When the oil is hot, add the merguez, breaking up any large pieces with a wooden spoon. Cook until the sausage is well browned, about 5 minutes, then add the asparagus mixture back in.

continued

6   When the pasta is done, use a slotted spoon to transfer it to the sauté pan with the merguez and asparagus, reserving the pasta water. Continue to cook over medium heat until a light, silky sauce forms. Add the lemon juice, and toss. If the pasta seems too dry, add some of the pasta water.

7   To serve, divide the pasta mixture between two bowls and season to taste with pepper. Spoon half of the ricotta on top of each bowl and sprinkle each with half of the bread crumbs.

Tuna Noodle Casserole

Leaving out the typical layer of cheese and salt-bomb of canned soup not only dramatically reduces the sodium in this comfort-food classic, but also makes it lighter while still being plenty flavorful.

You could bake this casserole in a separate baking dish, but I just use a Dutch oven for both the stovetop cooking and the baking, so there is one less dish to clean.

Makes: 4 servings
TOTAL SODIUM: 401 mg
SODIUM PER SERVING:
About 100 mg

½ pound fusilli or other short pasta
4 tablespoons unsalted butter, divided
½ medium onion, chopped
1 clove garlic, minced

4 button mushrooms, chopped
1 teaspoon fresh thyme leaves
¼ teaspoon dried sage
¼ teaspoon smoked paprika
Freshly ground black pepper
2 tablespoons all-purpose flour
1 cup whole milk

1 cup Chicken Stock (page 77)
Juice of ½ medium lemon
½ cup fresh or frozen peas
1 (2½-ounce) can unsalted albacore tuna in water, drained
½ cup bread crumbs (see page 52)

1   Fill a medium saucepot with water and bring to a boil over high heat. Add the pasta to the pot and cook until al dente according to the manufacturer's instructions, usually 10 to 12 minutes for dried pasta.

2   Drain in a colander, reserving ¾ cup of the pasta water, and set aside.

3   Preheat the oven to 350 degrees F.

continued

4   In a small Dutch oven over medium heat, melt 2 tablespoons of the butter. When the butter has melted, add the onion, garlic, mushrooms, thyme, sage, and paprika. Season to taste with pepper. Sauté until the onion has softened, about 5 minutes. Add the flour and cook until no dry bits remain, about 1 minute. Add the milk a little at a time, stirring constantly. Stir in the chicken stock and simmer until the sauce thickens to a creamy soup consistency, about 5 minutes. Add the lemon juice, peas, and tuna. Stir in the pasta and about ½ cup of the reserved pasta water. Stir, and add a little more pasta water if needed—it should be pretty saucy.

5   In a small bowl, mix the bread crumbs and remaining 2 tablespoons of butter. Sprinkle the mixture evenly across the top of the casserole and bake until the top is golden, about 25 minutes. Serve immediately.

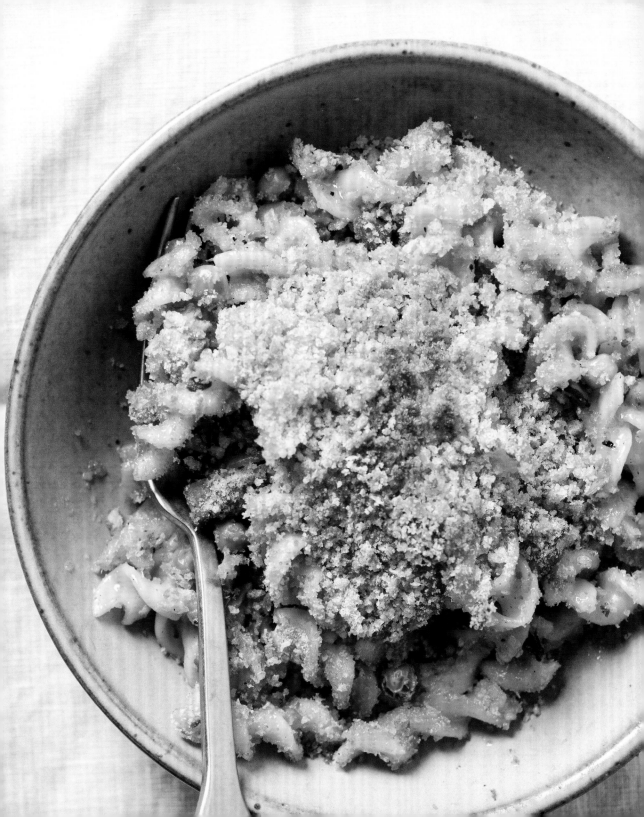

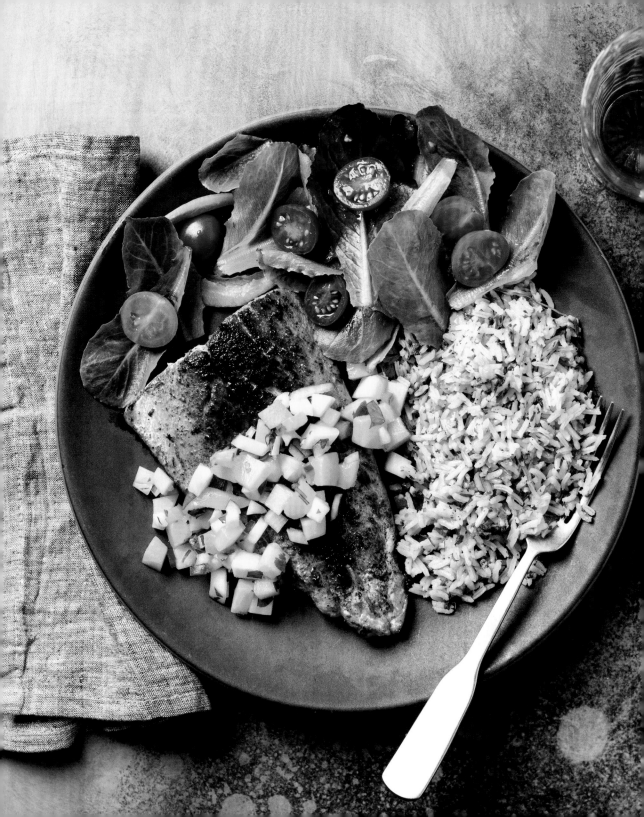

Salmon with Mango Salsa

Although quite simple to prepare, this salmon makes a really elegant meal, particularly served with the Dutch Oven Herbed Rice (page 216). Even though this is "blackened" salmon, you don't want to overcook it. A very hot pan will help achieve the perfect sear while keeping the center medium.

Makes: 2 servings

TOTAL SODIUM: 350 mg

SODIUM PER SERVING:
  About 175 mg

—————

2 salmon fillets, skin on, about ½ pound each

1 tablespoon olive oil

2 tablespoons Jerk Spice (page 40)

1 tablespoon unsalted butter

1 clove garlic, smashed

Juice of 1 medium lime

1 cup Mango Salsa (page 15)

1   Brush the salmon fillets with the olive oil, and sprinkle the jerk spice on both sides.

2   In a large skillet over medium-high heat, melt the butter. When the butter has melted, rub the garlic clove around the pan and save the garlic for another use. Increase the heat to high and add the fillets, skin side down. Cook for 3 minutes, and, using a spatula, carefully flip them. Cook until blackened, another 2 to 3 minutes.

3   To serve, transfer the salmon to two plates, pour the lime juice over the fillets, and top with the salsa.

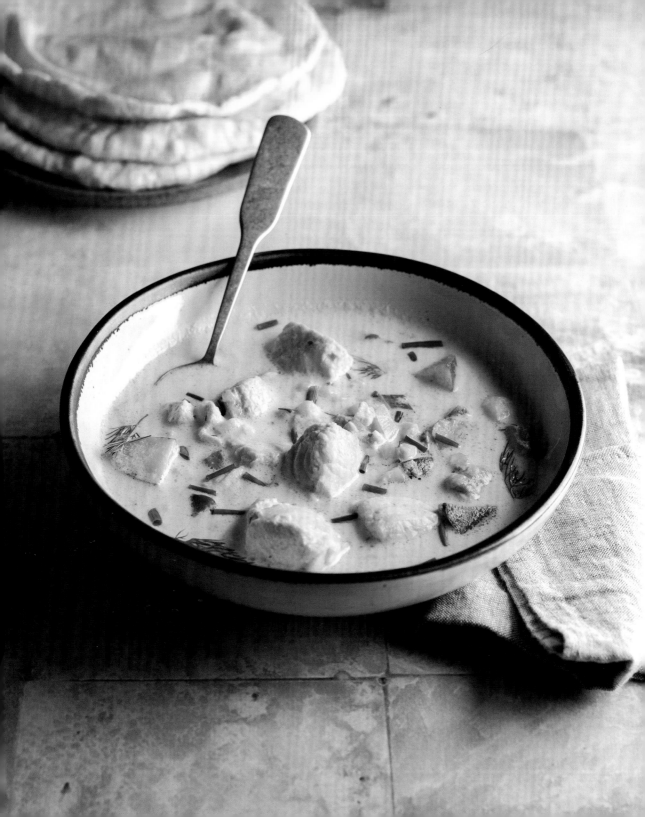

Salmon Chowder

Going low sodium, I didn't think I'd be able to enjoy chowder again. Clams, bacon, and dairy are all high in sodium, so all three combined usually means a bowl of chowder is off the charts. The canned version usually comes in around 800 milligrams per cup (and let's face it, it's not very often you only eat a cup). But by swapping out the clams for salmon and making a few other tweaks, this recipe is only a little over 800 milligrams for the whole hearty potful. If you aren't a big fan of salmon, you can swap in another fish, such as halibut or cod.

I use regular bacon, not the low-sodium kind, in this recipe and leave out the salt, so you get just a hint of the smoky, salty flavor indicative of most seafood chowders. Of course, you can use low-sodium Bacon (page 98) instead, but if you do, you'll probably want to add a bit of light salt.

Makes: 4 hearty servings

TOTAL SODIUM: 852 mg

SODIUM PER SERVING:
About 213 mg

½ pound new potatoes, quartered
1 strip uncured bacon
2 cups whole milk
1 cup heavy cream
1 bunch green onions, trimmed and chopped
1 cup fresh corn kernels
2 cloves garlic, minced

1 bay leaf
1 teaspoon fresh thyme leaves
½ teaspoon red pepper flakes
1 tablespoon all-purpose flour
½ cup Chicken Stock (page 77) or Vegetable Broth (page 79)
1 (12-ounce) salmon fillet, cut into 1-inch cubes

2 teaspoons freshly squeezed lemon juice
1 teaspoon chopped fresh dill
1 teaspoon chopped fresh flat-leaf parsley leaves
Freshly ground black pepper
A few fresh chives, for garnish

continued

1   Put the potatoes in a medium pot and fill with water to cover. Bring the water to a boil over medium-high heat. Cook until the potatoes are tender, about 8 minutes. Drain in a colander and set aside.

2   Meanwhile, in a medium heavy-bottomed pot over medium heat, fry the bacon, flipping it once, until crisp, about 5 minutes. Remove it from the pot, crumble it onto a plate, and set aside.

3   While the bacon cooks, combine the milk and cream in a small pot and heat on low until warm to the touch, about 4 minutes.

4   In the same pot used to cook the bacon, add the green onions, corn, garlic, bay leaf, thyme, red pepper flakes, and flour. Sauté over medium heat until softened, about 5 minutes, then stir in the stock. Slowly add the warmed milk and cream. Bring to a gentle simmer (but do not boil), then stir in the potatoes, bacon, and salmon. Simmer until the salmon is cooked through, about another 8 minutes. Remove the bay leaf. Stir in the lemon juice, dill, and parsley. Season to taste with black pepper and garnish with the chives. Serve immediately.

Vegetarian Bolognese

The first time I made Marcella Hazan's classic and utterly delicious Bolognese sauce, I made a typical rookie mistake and didn't read through the time the recipe takes. It's ground beef, how long can it take to make? Well, as it turns out, "at least" four hours. Oops. Dinner was late that night.

You won't have that trouble with this veggie version, which takes less than an hour to make and is much lower in sodium than the traditional sauce but is still as hearty. It's the perfect low-sodium, meatless Monday night dinner.

Makes: 4 servings
TOTAL SODIUM: 358 mg
TOTAL PER SERVING:
About 90 mg

⅓ cup Le Puy lentils
2 tablespoons olive oil
1 medium onion, chopped
¼ teaspoon light salt
½ teaspoon red pepper flakes
2 cloves garlic, minced
1 medium carrot, minced

1 bay leaf
8 ounces cremini, shiitake, or portobello mushrooms, finely minced into ⅛-inch pieces
3 tablespoons tomato paste
½ cup dry white wine
1 (14-ounce) can unsalted crushed or chopped tomatoes

Pinch of freshly grated nutmeg
2 tablespoons heavy cream, half-and-half, or whole milk
½ pound bucatini or other long pasta
¼ cup chopped fresh flat-leaf parsley leaves, for garnish

1   In a small saucepan, cover the lentils with water and bring to a boil over medium-high heat. Reduce the heat to medium and simmer until al dente, about 20 minutes. Drain in a colander and set aside.

2   In a large, heavy-bottomed pot, heat the oil over medium-high heat. When the oil is shimmering, reduce the heat to medium and add the onion and salt. Cook until the onion starts to soften, about 5 minutes. Stir in the red pepper flakes, garlic, carrot, bay leaf, and 1 tablespoon of water. Cook until fragrant, about 10 minutes.

continued

3   Stir in the mushrooms and continue to cook, stirring about once every minute, until the mushrooms have given up their liquid, about 5 minutes. Stir in the lentils and tomato paste. Cook, stirring frequently, until all the vegetables are browned and softened, about another 10 minutes.

4   Stir in the wine and use a wooden spoon to loosen any brown bits in the bottom of the pot. Stir in the tomatoes and nutmeg, and cook until hot, another 5 minutes. Reduce the heat to low, remove the bay leaf, stir in the cream, and let the sauce simmer while the pasta cooks.

5   Fill a medium saucepot with water and bring to a boil over high heat. Add the pasta to the pot and cook until al dente according to the manufacturer's instructions, usually about 10 to 12 minutes for dried pasta.

6   Drain in a colander, reserving ¾ cup of the pasta water. Add the pasta to the sauce, along with about ½ cup of the reserved pasta water. Gently stir to coat the pasta with the sauce, adding a little more pasta water if needed.

7   Garnish with the parsley and serve immediately.

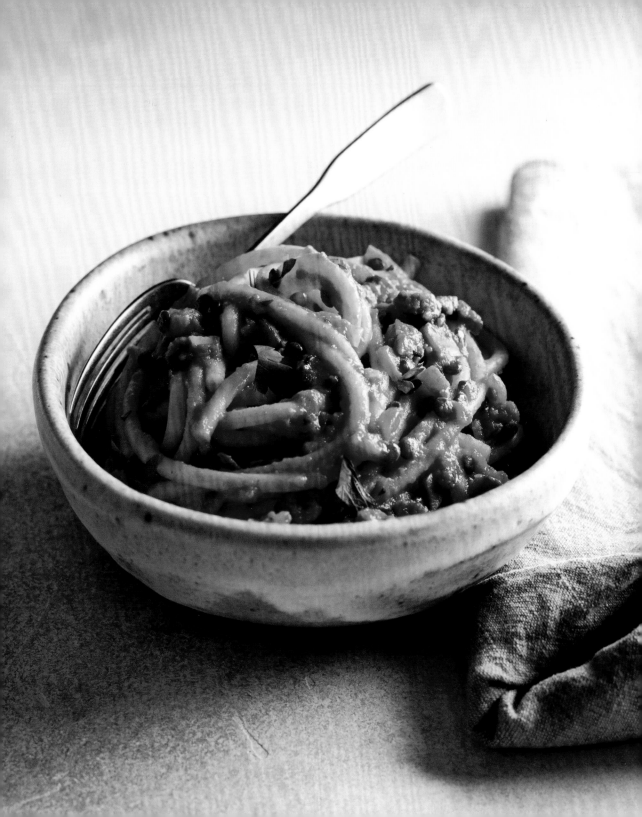

Ratatouille

Ratatouille recipes typically involve a lot of careful layering. Most nights, I don't have the patience for that. This rustic vegetable stew is just as delicious without the fussiness. Serve it with slices of crusty Baguette (page 49) for a hearty and healthy meal.

Makes: 8 servings
TOTAL SODIUM: 98 mg
SODIUM PER SERVING:
About 12 mg

2 tablespoons olive oil, divided
1 medium red onion, diced
4 cloves garlic, sliced
1 red or yellow bell pepper, diced
½ Anaheim chili, stemmed, seeded, and thinly sliced
1 pound butternut or other winter squash, peeled, seeded, and diced
1 medium zucchini (about ⅓ pound), diced
1 medium eggplant (about 1 pound), diced
1 cup cooked Chickpeas (page 82)
2 plum tomatoes, diced
1 tablespoon tomato paste
1 tablespoon fresh basil leaves
1 teaspoon granulated sugar
Freshly ground black pepper
¼ cup fresh cilantro leaves, for garnish
¼ cup fresh basil, for garnish

1   Preheat the oven to 400 degrees F.

2   In a 4-quart Dutch oven or other heavy pot with a lid, heat 1 tablespoon of the oil over medium heat. When the oil is hot, add the onion and sauté until it is softened, about 5 minutes. Add the garlic, bell pepper, and chili, and sauté until softened, about 5 minutes. Add the squash and sauté until softened, another 5 minutes. Transfer the vegetables to a bowl and set aside.

3   Heat the remaining tablespoon of oil in the Dutch oven over medium heat. When it is hot, add the zucchini and eggplant and sauté until softened, about 5 minutes. Return the onion mixture to the pot, and stir in the chickpeas, tomatoes, tomato paste, basil, sugar, and ½ cup of water. Cover and transfer to the oven. Roast for 30 minutes, then remove the lid. Roast for another 15 minutes, until the vegetables are slightly caramelized on top.

4   To serve, season to taste with black pepper, and garnish with the cilantro and basil.

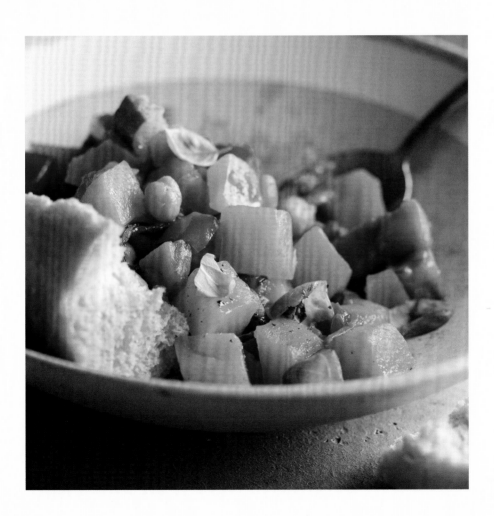

Butternut Squash Curry

Pumpkin curry may not be on the menu at your Thai takeout joint, but pumpkin is a traditional Thai food and makes a great curry. I use butternut squash because it is less watery than most winter squashes. You could also use kabocha when it's in season.

Makes: 4 servings
TOTAL SODIUM: 302 mg
SODIUM PER SERVING:
  About 76 mg

3 tablespoons olive oil, divided
1 pound butternut or other winter squash, peeled, seeded, and cubed
¼ teaspoon light salt

1 medium yellow onion, diced
½ teaspoon yellow or brown mustard seeds
½ teaspoon cumin seeds
2 cloves garlic, minced
1 teaspoon ground coriander
½ teaspoon ground turmeric

2 jalapeño or serrano chilies, seeded and chopped
1 cup water
1 cup full-fat coconut milk
2 tablespoons freshly squeezed lime juice
Cilantro leaves, for garnish

1   In a large skillet over medium-high heat, heat add 2 tablespoons of the oil. When the oil is hot, add the squash and cook, stirring occasionally, until browned on all sides, about 4 minutes. Stir in the salt. Transfer the squash to a bowl and set aside.

2   Heat the remaining tablespoon of oil in the skillet over medium heat. When the oil is hot, add the onion and mustard and cumin seeds. Cook for about 1 minute. Add the garlic, coriander, turmeric, and chilies. Cook for 1 more minute. Return the squash to the skillet and add the water. Simmer until the squash is tender, about 15 minutes. Add the coconut milk and simmer until warmed through, about 10 minutes more.

3   Stir in the lime juice just before serving, and garnish with the cilantro.

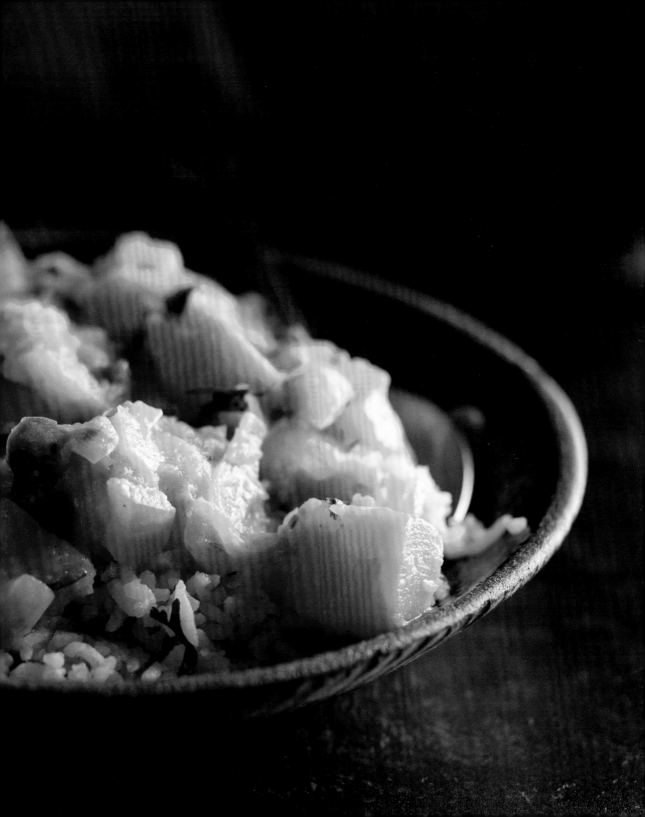

Sides

Lemon Brown Butter Cauliflower Bake

Lemon, sage, and brown butter make a delightful palette of flavors for this simple baked cauliflower, but you can also add some "mix-ins" for variety—try toasted pine nuts, rehydrated raisins or currants, or cubes of lightly roasted apple.

Makes: 2 servings
TOTAL SODIUM: 400 mg
SODIUM PER SERVING:
    About 200 mg

2 tablespoons olive oil
6 fresh sage leaves

Zest and juice of ½
    medium lemon
¼ teaspoon red pepper
    flakes (optional)
Tiny pinch of light salt
1 cup whole milk
Pinch of fresh nutmeg

Large pinch of freshly
    ground black pepper
1 head cauliflower (about
    1 pound), cut into
    florets
2 tablespoons unsalted
    butter, cut into pieces

1   Heat the oil in a small skillet over medium heat until it sizzles when you touch it with a sage leaf. Fry the sage leaves, stirring, until they are fragrant and crisp, only about 1 minute. (Be careful not to burn them.) Transfer them to a paper towel to cool.

2   Once the sage leaves have cooled, crumble them into a small bowl, along with the lemon zest, red pepper flakes, and salt. Mix well and set aside.

3   Preheat the oven to 400 degrees F.

4   In a medium saucepan over medium-high heat, combine the milk, 1 cup of water, and the nutmeg, and bring to a simmer. Add the cauliflower, reduce the heat to low, and cover. Cook until the cauliflower is barely tender, about 15 minutes. The milk will likely curdle, but don't worry! Any little milk bits clinging to the florets will just make them that much tastier.

continued

5   Drain the cauliflower well in a colander over the sink, and transfer it to a small casserole dish. Bake until it is lightly golden, about 20 minutes.

6   Meanwhile, in a small, light-colored skillet over medium heat, melt the butter. Cook, stirring frequently, until the foam subsides, the butter is golden brown, and the solids have separated and turned a toasty brown, about 5 minutes. Remove the skillet from the heat and stir in the lemon juice.

7   Pour the butter over the baked cauliflower and stir to coat. Sprinkle with the reserved sage mixture and serve.

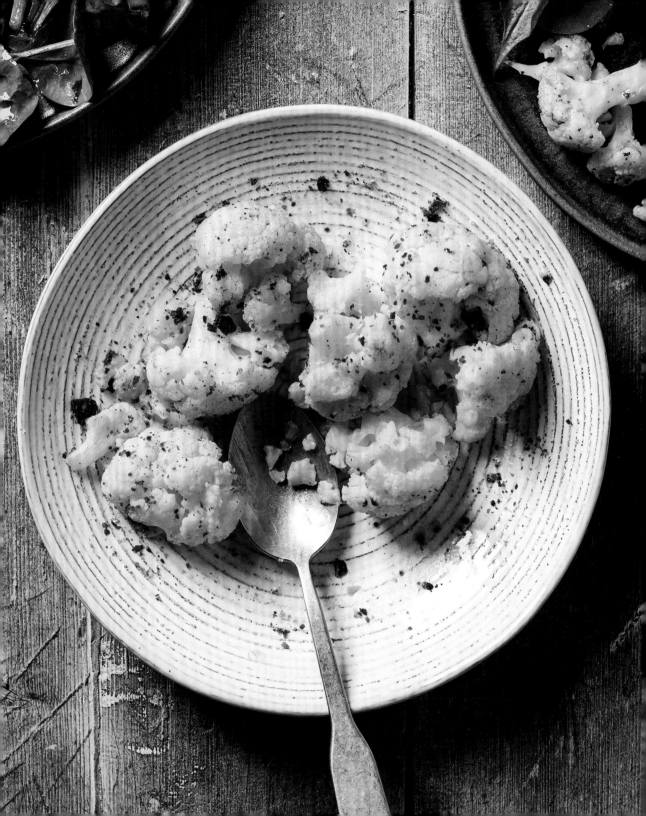

Blistered Cherry Tomatoes

This is a showstopping side dish that I love to serve in all sorts of ways. The tomatoes make a great toast topping or a delicious garnish on Chèvre (page 107) or Ricotta (page 105). Or you could just eat them by themselves in a big bowl with a spoon. The roasting brings out even more sweetness from already sweet cherry tomatoes.

Makes: 4 servings
TOTAL SODIUM: 152 mg
SODIUM PER SERVING:
   About 38 mg
_____

1 pint cherry tomatoes
Zest of 1 medium lemon
1 clove garlic, minced
1 tablespoon olive oil

1 teaspoon fresh thyme
   leaves
1 teaspoon chopped
   fresh rosemary leaves
½ teaspoon red pepper
   flakes
½ teaspoon light brown
   sugar

2 teaspoons chopped
   fresh flat-leaf parsley
   leaves
⅛ teaspoon light salt
Freshly ground black
   pepper

1   Preheat the oven to 425 degrees F.

2   In a medium bowl, toss the tomatoes with the lemon zest, garlic, oil, thyme, rosemary, red pepper flakes, and sugar. Transfer the tomatoes to a small casserole dish.

3   Roast for 20 minutes, then switch to the broiler and broil until the tops of the tomatoes are lightly charred, about 5 minutes. Remove from the oven and sprinkle with the parsley and salt. Season to taste with black pepper.

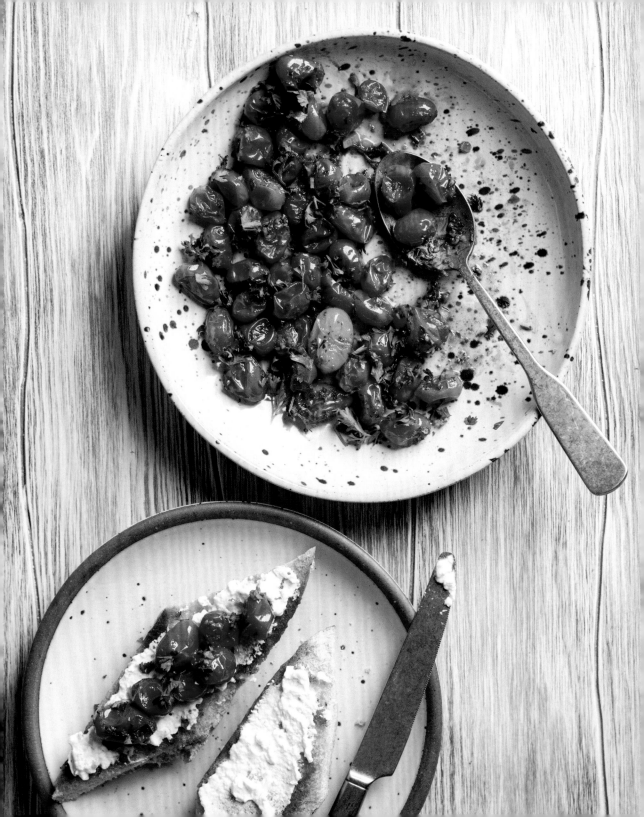

Spaghetti Squash with Caramelized Onions

I get a weekly "ugly" food box that has a mix of whatever farmers grew too much of or a distributor found unsellable. For about four weeks in a row earlier this year, each box had a spaghetti squash, and each week, I struggled to find a way to prepare it that made me happy.

Then I stumbled on a few recipes for spaghetti squash with caramelized onions, but most loaded up on the cheese. I started playing around with them, and this recipe emerged. Now I can't wait for the next spaghetti squash to show up in my box!

Makes: 4 servings
TOTAL SODIUM: 258 mg
SODIUM PER SERVING:
   About 65 mg

---

1 (3-pound) spaghetti
   squash
2 tablespoons olive oil,
   divided

1 medium onion, roughly
   chopped
1 clove garlic, minced
1 teaspoon fresh
   rosemary
1 cup stemmed, chopped
   kale
Zest and juice of 1
   medium lemon

2 tablespoons heavy
   cream
1 teaspoon fresh thyme
   leaves
Freshly ground black
   pepper
Aleppo pepper or other
   chili flakes

1   Preheat the oven to 350 degrees F. Line a baking sheet with parchment paper.

2   Cut the spaghetti squash in half and remove the seeds. Brush both halves all over with 1 tablespoon of the oil, and place them cut side down on the baking sheet. Roast until the cut side is lightly golden and the interior is fork-tender, about 45 minutes.

3   Meanwhile, in a large skillet over medium-low heat, heat the remaining table-spoon of oil. When the oil is hot, add the onion. Cook, stirring occasionally, until it is soft and translucent, about 15 minutes. Add the garlic and rosemary, and continue to cook until the onions have caramelized to a deep golden brown, another 15 minutes. Add a splash of water if the mixture gets too dry and starts to burn. Add the kale, increase the heat to medium, and cook until the kale has softened, about 3 minutes. Remove from the heat and cover.

4   When the squash has finished roasting, remove it from the oven and let it cool slightly. When it is cool enough to handle, use a fork to scrape out and shred the squash into a serving bowl. Add the squash, zest and juice, cream, and thyme to the onion mixture, mixing well. Season to taste with black and Aleppo pepper.

Spiced Roasted Carrots

I like to use medium-size carrots, left whole, for this recipe. A little less than an inch thick at their thickest is about the right width for the perfect caramelization and bite. If you are using thicker carrots, cut them on the bias into smaller pieces after the first roast, before you add them to the butter mixture.

Makes: 4 servings

TOTAL SODIUM: 498 mg

SODIUM PER SERVING:
   About 125 mg

1½ pounds carrots,
   trimmed and peeled
1 tablespoon olive oil
½ teaspoon cumin seeds

1 tablespoon Harissa
   (page 8)
1 tablespoon unsalted
   butter, melted
2 teaspoons white wine
   vinegar
1 teaspoon honey

Freshly ground black
   pepper
½ cup toasted and
   chopped unsalted
   almonds, pistachios, or
   other nuts (optional)
½ cup pomegranate
   seeds (optional)

1   Preheat the oven to 475 degrees F, and line a baking sheet with parchment paper.

2   Spread the carrots on the baking sheet and drizzle with the olive oil, tossing a little bit to coat each carrot in the oil. Roast until they are dark brown in spots, but still have a little bite to them, 12 to 14 minutes. Remove from the oven and set aside.

3   Reduce the heat to 300 degrees.

4   In a large bowl, combine the cumin seeds, harissa, butter, vinegar, and honey. Put the carrots in the bowl, stir to coat them with the butter mixture, and let them marinate for 5 minutes.

5   Return the carrots to the baking sheet, and roast until completely tender, 5 to 7 minutes. Season to taste with pepper and toss with the nuts and pomegranate seeds. Serve warm.

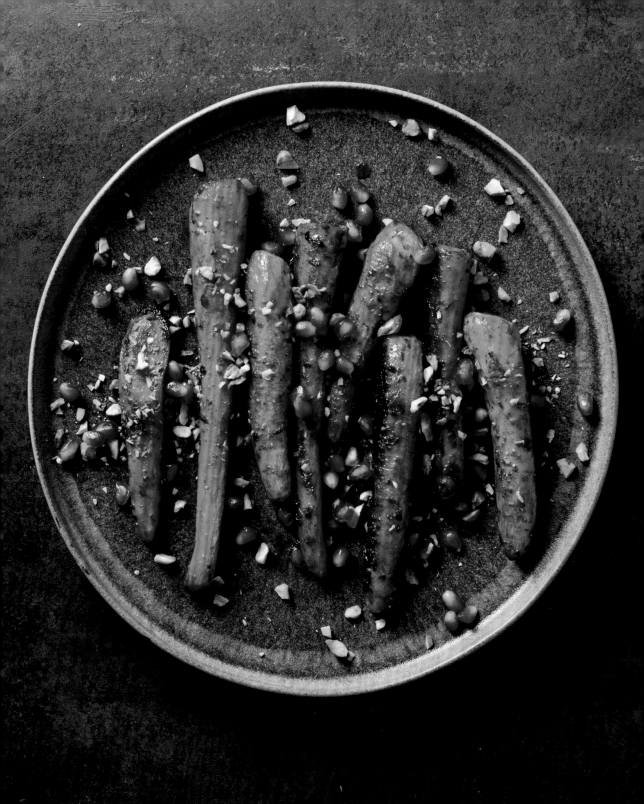

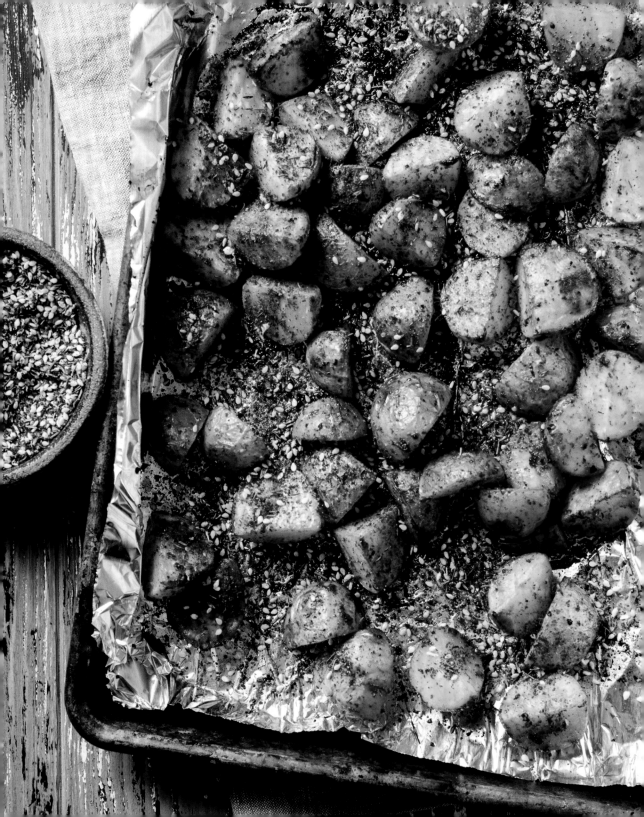

Roasted Potatoes with Za'atar

Fingerling potatoes come in all shapes, sizes, and even colors. Russian Banana fingerlings, a waxy yellow oblong type, are one of the most common, but if you purchase a mixed bag, you'll probably also get some Purple Peruvian and Ruby Crescents as well. They are all delicious!

To make sure they cook evenly, cut any larger potatoes into smaller pieces, so the potatoes are roughly the same size. Adding the za'atar near the end of the cooking toasts it slightly without burning it, so the flavor is at its best.

Makes: 4 servings
TOTAL SODIUM: 96 mg
SODIUM PER SERVING:
   About 24 mg
——————
1 pound fingerling
   potatoes, cut to equal
   size if needed

1 tablespoon olive oil,
   plus more for drizzling
Juice of ½ medium
   lemon

1 tablespoon piment
   d'Espelette or other
   chili flakes
2 tablespoons Za'atar
   (page 41)

1   Preheat the oven to 400 degrees F. Line a baking sheet with parchment paper.

2   In a medium bowl, toss the potatoes with the oil, lemon juice, and piment d'Espelette. Spread the potatoes out on the baking sheet, and roast they are until golden brown, crisp on the outside, and soft in the middle, 30 to 40 minutes.

3   Pull them out of the oven, drizzle a bit of oil over them, and sprinkle the za'atar on top. Stir to coat them evenly, and return them to the oven for another 5 minutes. Serve immediately.

Crispy Sweet Potato Wedges

Unsalted fries are a bummer, so these seasoned, roasted sweet potato wedges really save the day. Be sure to keep an eye on them while they bake: a few charred bits are great, but you don't want to go overboard.

Makes: 2 servings

TOTAL SODIUM: 256 mg

SODIUM PER SERVING:
About 128 mg

1 teaspoon cornstarch

1 teaspoon garlic powder

1 teaspoon smoked paprika

½ teaspoon red pepper flakes

1 pound sweet potatoes, peeled and cut into ½-inch-thick wedges

¼ cup olive oil

Freshly ground black pepper

1   Put the potatoes in a medium pot and cover them with water. Bring to a boil over high heat, then reduce the heat to low and simmer until they are slightly soft, about 10 minutes. Drain them well in a colander.

2   Meanwhile, preheat the oven to 400 degrees F and line a baking sheet with aluminum foil.

3   In a medium bowl, combine the cornstarch, garlic powder, paprika, and red pepper flakes.

4   Pour the oil on the baking sheet and place it in the oven for 5 minutes to heat the oil.

5   Toss the potatoes in the spice mixture. Carefully remove the baking sheet from the oven and spread the potatoes on it. Bake them for 20 minutes on one side, then flip the potatoes with a spatula and bake them on the second side until they are crisp, another 15 minutes.

6   Season to taste with black pepper and serve immediately.

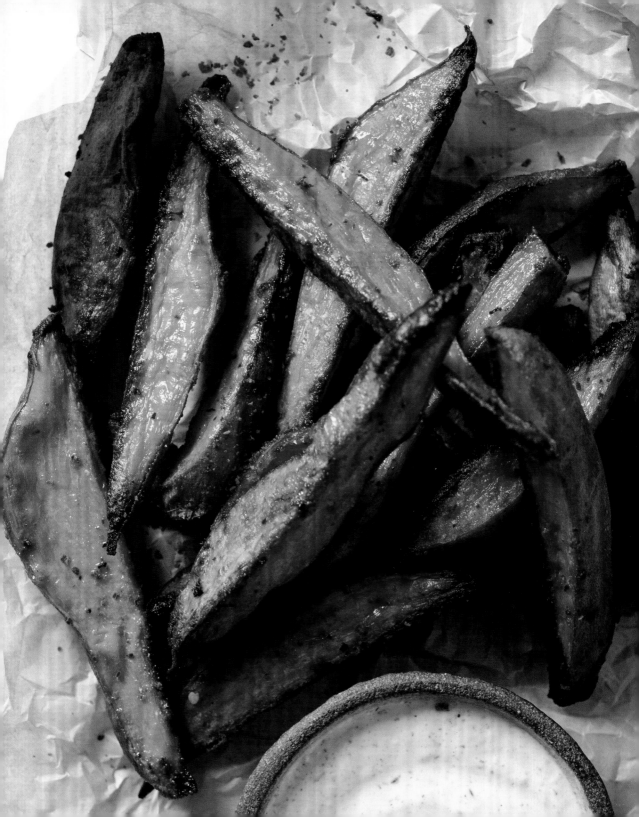

Dutch Oven Herbed Rice

The website Food52 is one of my go-to sources for recipes, and its cookbook *Food52 A New Way to Dinner* is a great one. That's where I learned the basics of this herby baked-rice dish, which I've reworked to make low sodium. It's packed with flavor and pairs well with a variety of cuisines. I serve it with roasts, tacos, chicken curry, or Salmon with Mango Salsa (page 191).

Makes: 6 servings

TOTAL SODIUM: 212 mg

SODIUM PER SERVING: About 35 mg

1 cup chopped cilantro leaves

1 cup chopped fresh flat-leaf parsley leaves

1 cup chopped fresh mint leaves

Zest of 1 medium lime

3 cloves garlic

1 jalapeño, stemmed and seeded

3 tablespoons olive oil, divided

¼ teaspoon freshly ground black pepper

1 bay leaf

1 medium onion, finely chopped

1 tablespoon plus 1 teaspoon red wine vinegar

3 cups water

⅛ teaspoon light salt

2 cups uncooked basmati rice

1   Preheat the oven to 350 degrees F.

2   In the bowl of a food processor, pulse the cilantro, parsley, mint, lime zest, garlic, and jalapeño to create a rough paste. (If you don't have a food processor, you can just finely chop each ingredient and mix them together.) Set aside.

3   In a small Dutch oven, heat 1 tablespoon of the oil over medium heat. When the oil is hot, add the black pepper and bay leaf, and cook for 2 minutes. Add the onion and cook until soft and translucent, 8 to 10 minutes.

4   When the onion has softened, add half of the herb paste. Mix the remaining herb paste with the vinegar and remaining 2 tablespoons olive oil and set aside.

5 Add the water and salt. Increase the heat to high and bring to a boil. Stir in the rice and bring back to a boil. Cover, transfer the pot to the oven, and bake for 20 minutes undisturbed (do not remove the lid).

6 When the rice has cooked, discard the bay leaf, and fluff the rice with a fork. Stir in the remaining herb paste. If not serving immediately, re-cover the rice until ready to serve.

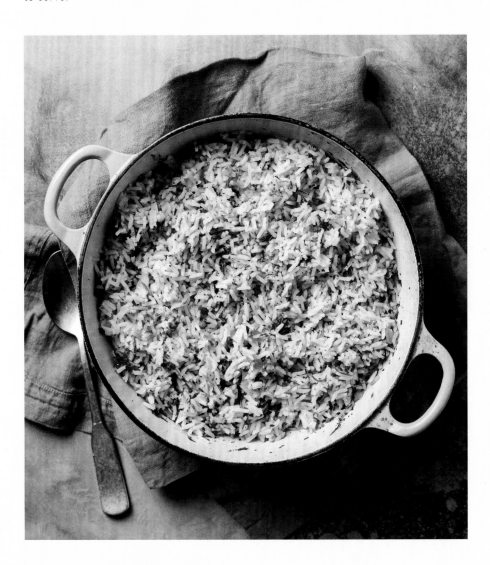

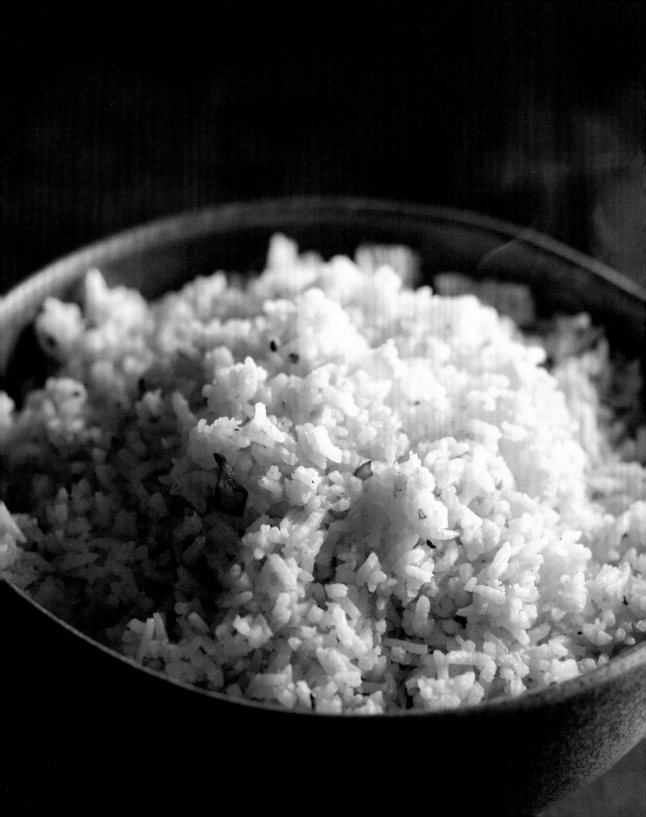

Spiced Basmati Rice

Plain white rice is a fine side dish, but this spiced rice isn't much harder to make and is a welcome change. The mixture of clove, cardamom, cinnamon, cumin, and mustard make it a natural accompaniment for Chicken Chana Masala (page 160) or Butternut Squash Curry (page 200). Using whole cinnamon, cloves, and cardamom keeps the flavors from these spices subtle.

Makes: 4 servings

TOTAL SODIUM: 36 mg

SODIUM PER SERVING:
  About 9 mg

———

2 cups uncooked long-grain basmati rice

2 whole cloves

2 cardamom pods

1 (2-inch) piece cinnamon stick

2 tablespoons unsalted butter

½ teaspoon brown mustard seeds

½ teaspoon cumin seeds

¼ teaspoon red pepper flakes

¼ teaspoon freshly ground black pepper

1 medium onion, chopped

½ teaspoon freshly grated ginger

¼ teaspoon turmeric

1   Put the rice in a medium bowl and cover with cool water. Let sit for at least 15 minutes, then drain in a colander.

2   If you are using a multicooker, put the rice and 2 cups of water in the pot, along with the cloves, cardamom pods, and cinnamon stick. Cover, being sure to set the steam vent to closed, and cook on high pressure for 6 minutes. Let the steam release naturally, which will take about 10 minutes (do not open the release valve).

3   If you are cooking the rice on the stovetop, in a heavy-bottomed medium saucepan with a tight-fitting lid, bring 3 cups of water to a boil. Add the rice, cloves, cardamom pods, and cinnamon stick, and return to a boil. When the water is boiling, cover the pan, and reduce the heat to the lowest setting. Let the rice cook for 15 minutes, then turn off the heat and let it sit, covered, for another 5 minutes.

continued

4   Remove and discard the cloves, cardamom pods, and cinnamon stick.

5   In a large skillet, heat the butter over medium heat. When the butter is no longer foaming, add the mustard and cumin seeds, red pepper flakes, and black pepper. Cook until the spices are fragrant, about 3 minutes, and then add the onion and ginger. Reduce the heat to medium-low, and sauté until the onions are golden, about 5 minutes.

6   Add the rice and turmeric and sauté until heated throughout, another 3 to 4 minutes.

7   Serve immediately or cover and keep warm for up to 20 minutes before serving. If you have leftovers, place a moist paper towel over the bowl when reheating in the microwave for the best results.

Vegetable Fried Rice

Pick and choose your own veggies to throw into this fried rice—it's a great recipe for cleaning out the fridge. I like bok choy, broccoli, and snow peas, but you could add carrot, green peas, celery, or whatever you have on hand. You'll want about 5 cups of chopped vegetables total.

Makes: 4 servings
TOTAL SODIUM: 768 mg
SODIUM PER SERVING:
About 192 mg

1 large egg
2 tablespoons sunflower
  or other vegetable oil
1 medium onion, diced
1 red bell pepper, diced
2 cups chopped broccoli
  florets (about 1
  medium head)

1 cup chopped bok choy
1 cup snow peas
1 cup sliced mushrooms
2 cloves garlic, minced
Zest of 1 medium lemon
1 tablespoon minced
  ginger
4 cups cooled cooked
  plain steamed rice
½ cup chopped green
  onions

¼ cup chopped fresh
  cilantro leaves
2 tablespoons coconut
  aminos
1 tablespoon toasted
  sesame oil
1 tablespoon unseasoned
  rice vinegar
Red pepper flakes

1   In a small bowl, lightly beat the egg. Set aside.

2   In a wok or large sauté pan, heat 1 tablespoon of the oil over high heat. When the oil is hot and shimmering, add the onion and bell pepper, and stir-fry until the onion softens, about 3 minutes. Add the broccoli, bok choy, and snow peas and stir-fry until heated through, another 5 minutes. Use a slotted spoon to remove the vegetables to a plate. Set aside.

continued

3   Add the remaining tablespoon of oil, and when shimmering, add the mushrooms and stir-fry until they have given up their liquid, about 5 minutes. Add the garlic, lemon zest, and ginger, and stir-fry for about 1 minute. Add the rice, and stir until there are no clumps, about 2 minutes. Push the rice aside to make a well in the center of the wok. Add the beaten egg, and cook, lightly stirring without integrating into the rice, until most of the egg is solid. Then stir it into the rice.

4   Return the vegetables to the wok, thoroughly combining them with the rice. Stir in the green onions, cilantro, coconut aminos, sesame oil, and vinegar. Season to taste with red pepper flakes. Serve warm.

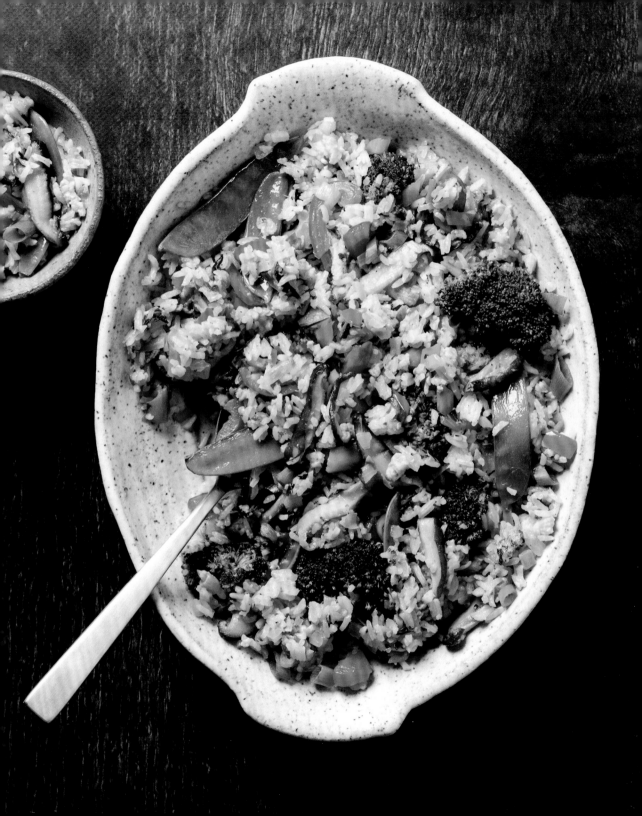

Desserts

Brown Butter Chocolate Chip Cookies

Sodium-free baking soda browns a little differently than traditional baking soda, which changes the caramelization point of sugar due to its alkalinity. To make up for that, this recipe uses dark brown sugar and brown butter to achieve traditional-looking cookies (along with a great flavor boost).

Chocolate is a no-no if you are limiting caffeine, so if that's the case for you, try making these with carob or dried fruit (dried cherries or cranberries are excellent). But if you can tolerate a small amount of chocolate, these are the perfect indulgence. My preference is at least 72 percent dark chocolate.

Makes: 2 dozen cookies

TOTAL SODIUM: 473 mg

SODIUM PER COOKIE:
About 20 mg

1 cup (2 sticks) unsalted butter, cut into pieces

2¾ cups (330 grams) all-purpose flour

2 teaspoons sodium-free baking soda

¼ teaspoon light salt

2 cups (400 grams) lightly packed dark brown sugar

¼ cup granulated sugar

2 large eggs

2 teaspoons vanilla extract

5 ounces chocolate of choice, coarsely chopped

1 cup coarsely chopped unsalted toasted nuts (optional)

1   Line two baking sheets with parchment paper.

2   In a medium, light-colored skillet, melt the butter over medium heat, and cook, stirring frequently, until the foam subsides, the butter is golden brown, and the solids have separated and turned a toasty brown, about 5 minutes.

3   In a medium bowl, combine the flour, baking soda, and salt.

continued

4   In the bowl of a stand mixer fitted with the paddle attachment, beat the brown butter and both sugars on medium speed until combined, about 1 minute. Scrape down the sides of the bowl. Add 1 of the eggs and mix on low until it is well incorporated. Scrape down the bowl again. Add the remaining egg and the vanilla. Mix until it is well incorporated and the mixture is lighter in color, 1 minute more. Scrape down the bowl once more.

5   Add the flour mixture and mix on low until just combined, about 30 seconds. Fold in the chocolate and nuts with a spatula or spoon.

6   Drop the dough by heaping tablespoons onto one of the baking sheets. Don't let them touch, but they can be very close together (the spacing doesn't matter because you'll be chilling the dough). Chill the dough in the freezer for 30 minutes or in the refrigerator for 2 hours, until firm.

7   If you'll be baking the cookies right away, preheat the oven to 350 degrees F about halfway through the chilling time. If you plan on baking the cookies at a later time, after the dough has chilled, transfer it to a ziplock freezer bag and store in the freezer for up to 3 months. The cookies can be baked without defrosting.

8   Distribute the dough balls on the baking sheets, leaving at least ½ inch between each. Bake for 12 minutes (13 minutes if baking from frozen), or until the cookies are just lightly golden on the outside. If you bake both sheets at the same time, place them on separate racks and rotate the sheets after 5 minutes. Cool the cookies on the baking sheet for 5 minutes, then transfer them to a wire rack to cool completely.

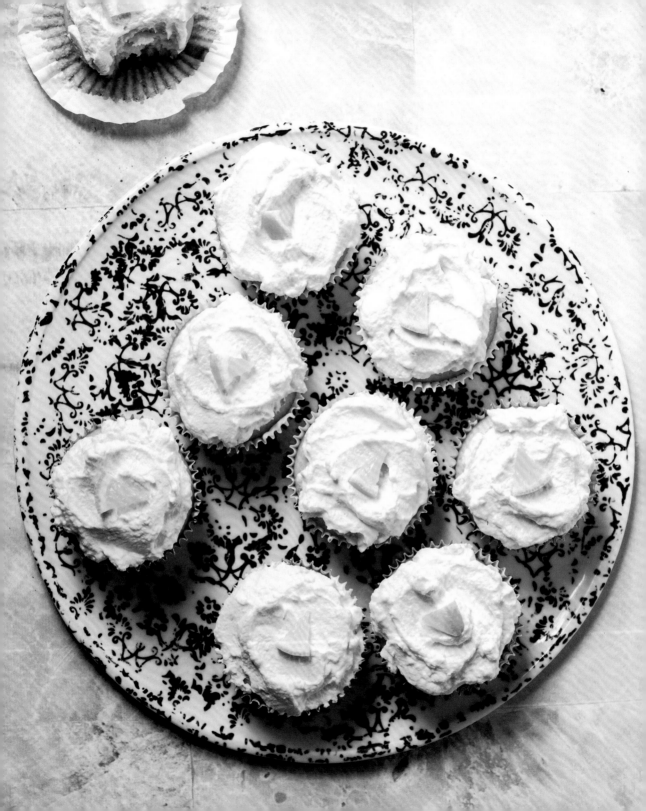

Lemon Cupcakes

I am not a fan of cupcakes that have more frosting than cake, particularly when that frosting is a dense block of sugared butter. I always end up scraping most of it off to enjoy the cake beneath. These lemon cupcakes are frosted with a subtly sweet lemon whipped cream, which is like eating a lemon cloud. No scraping needed.

These cupcakes must be completely cooled before frosting, so be sure to allow enough time. And because the lemon cream is wetter than buttercream frosting and doesn't hold up as long, you won't be able to frost these ahead of time—you'll need to wait until just before serving.

Makes: 18 cupcakes
TOTAL SODIUM: 726 mg
SODIUM PER CUPCAKE:
   About 40 mg

_____

FOR THE CUPCAKES
1 recipe "Box" Yellow
   Cake Mix (page 74)
1 cup water
2 large eggs

¼ cup vegetable oil
½ teaspoon vanilla
   extract
Zest and juice of 2
   medium lemons

FOR THE FROSTING
2 cups heavy cream

6 tablespoons
   confectioners' sugar
Zest and juice of 1 large
   lemon
Thin lemon slices cut
   into triangles, or
   berries or edible
   flowers, for garnish

1   Preheat the oven to 350 degrees F.

2   Line two 12-cup standard muffin tins with 18 cupcake liners.

3   To make the cupcakes, in a large bowl combine the cake mix, water, eggs, oil, vanilla, and lemon zest and juice. Beat until smooth.

4   Spoon the batter into the tins, filling each cup about two-thirds full (a little less than ¼ cup each). Bake until the cupcakes are lightly golden, about 20 minutes, or until a skewer inserted into the center of a cupcake comes out clean.

continued

5   Remove the cupcakes from the pan and transfer to a wire rack to cool completely.

6   To make the lemon cream frosting, using a hand mixer or a stand mixer fitted with the whisk attachment, beat the cream until it begins to thicken, about 1 minute. Add the sugar and lemon juice and zest. Beat until fluffy, about 30 seconds. If the whipped cream starts to look grainy, stop beating and stir in 1 tablespoon or so of heavy cream—this should smooth it out.

7   Just before serving, pipe or spread the frosting on the cooled cupcakes and add the garnish.

Peach Cuppa Cuppa Stikka Buckle

This easiest of cake batters (which gets its name from the simple measurements of a cup of flour, a cup of sugar, and a stick of butter) is poured into a pan and layered with ripe fruit that sinks into the cake when baked. I like it best with peaches and a handful of blueberries or blackberries, but you can make it with a combination of other fruits. Use ripe, juicy peaches—there's no need to peel them.

Note that you'll need a small (two-quart) baking dish—be sure not to use a larger one, or the buckle will be too thin.

Makes: About 6 servings

TOTAL SODIUM: 389 mg

SODIUM PER SERVING:
   About 65 mg

---

5 medium peaches, pitted and sliced

1 tablespoon freshly squeezed lemon juice

1 cup (200 grams) granulated sugar, divided

½ cup (1 stick) unsalted butter

1 cup (120 grams) all-purpose flour

1 teaspoon sodium-free baking powder

½ teaspoon ground cinnamon

¼ teaspoon light salt

1 cup whole milk

1 teaspoon vanilla extract

1 cup berries (optional)

1   In a large bowl, combine the peaches with the lemon juice and 1 tablespoon of the sugar. Set aside to macerate.

2   Meanwhile, preheat the oven to 350 degrees F and line a baking sheet with aluminum foil.

3   Melt the butter by putting it in a small baking dish while the oven is warming. Remove it from the oven when it is slightly brown, about 8 minutes (watch to make sure it does not burn). Set aside.

continued

4   In a medium bowl, whisk the flour, remaining sugar, baking powder, cinnamon, and salt together. Whisk in the milk and vanilla until smooth.

5   Swirl the butter around the pan and up the sides. Pour about half the batter into the pan (don't stir it into the butter). Top with the peach slices and any accumulated juices as well as the berries, then top with the remaining batter.

6   Place the baking dish on the foil-lined baking sheet and bake until golden brown and the edges are lightly crisped, about 1 hour. Let sit for about 10 minutes before serving warm.

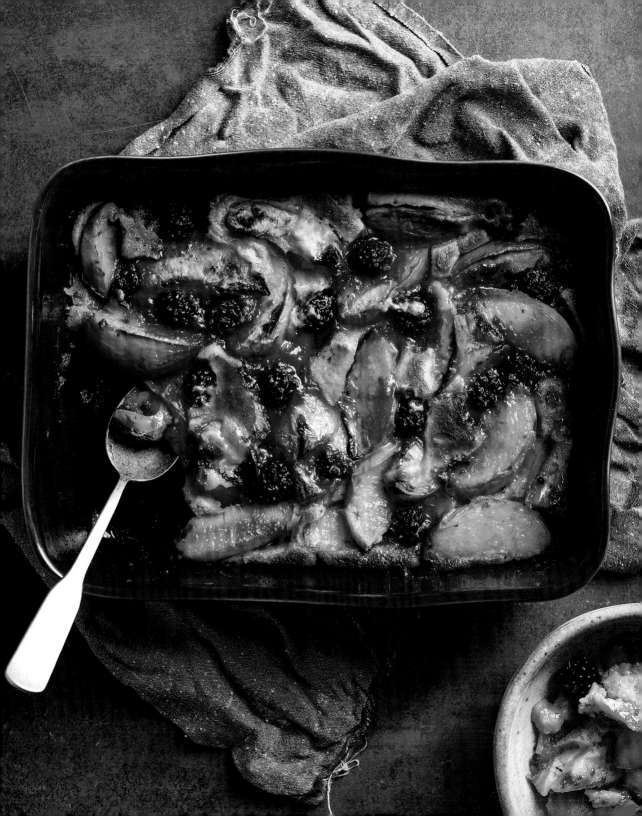

Butter Tarts

I had never heard of this classic Canadian pastry before I met my husband, but it instantly entered my dessert hall of fame. Since they're bite size, it's all too easy to eat two—or ten—of them, with their tender, flaky crust and caramelized, gooey filling.

Makes: 12 tarts

TOTAL SODIUM: 595 mg

SODIUM PER TART: About 50 mg

½ recipe Pie Dough (page 73)

¼ cup unsalted butter, room temperature

½ cup lightly packed light brown sugar

¼ cup light corn syrup

¼ cup dark corn syrup

½ teaspoon vanilla extract

¼ teaspoon light salt

1 large egg

⅔ cup raisins (optional)

1   On a generously floured work surface, roll the pie dough out to a little more than ¼ inch thick. Cut out 12 circles with a 3-inch biscuit cutter. (You will have leftover pastry—form it into a ball, wrap it in plastic wrap, and refrigerate or freeze it for another use.) Roll out each circle a bit more to make 4-inch rounds. Place each round into the cup of a muffin tin, using your fingers to gently press the dough to evenly cover the bottoms and sides of each cup. Refrigerate for at least 30 minutes and up to 12 hours.

2   Preheat the oven to 425 degrees F.

3   In the bowl of a stand mixer fitted with the paddle attachment (or in a medium bowl and using a hand mixer), cream the butter until it is soft. Add the brown sugar, both corn syrups, vanilla, and salt, scraping down the sides of the bowl as needed. Beat in the egg, then fold in the raisins.

4   Spoon about 1 tablespoon of the filling into the tart shells (they should be about half full). Place the muffin tin on a baking sheet, and bake until the sugar is bubbly and the crust is golden, 15 to 20 minutes. Some of the filling may bubble up and run over the side—that's OK.

5   Run a knife or offset spatula around the sides of the tin to loosen the tarts. Let them cool in the tin for at least 15 minutes before carefully releasing them. Remove them to a wire rack to cool to room temperature.

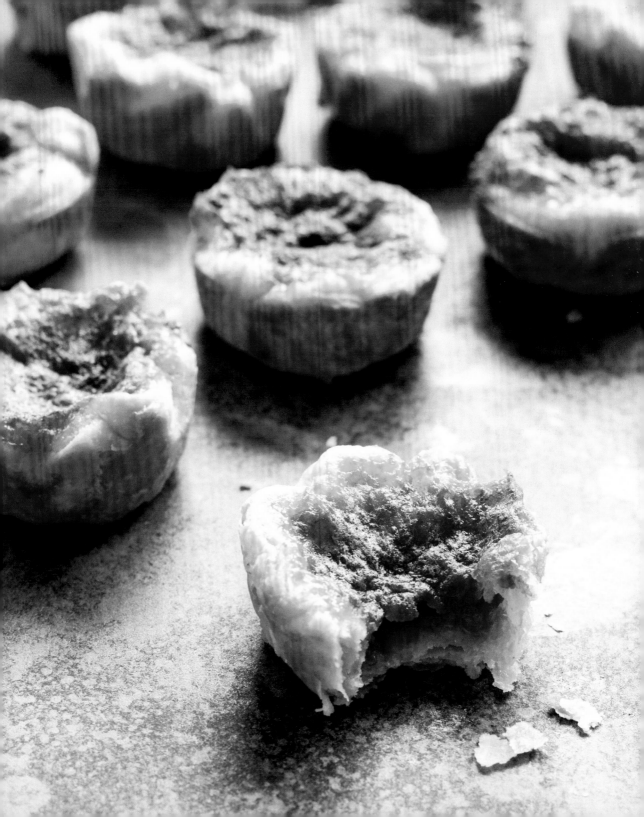

Pumpkin Slab Pie

I don't go pumpkin-spice crazy in the fall, but I do love a good slice of pumpkin pie now and then. I think pumpkin pie works particularly well in slab form because it's easier to slice and serve for a crowd. If the pastry-garnish pieces are too twee for you, just cut the excess pastry into strips, sprinkle them with a little cinnamon and sugar, and you'll have a great snack while you're waiting for the pie to cool.

This slab pie uses the same amount of pastry as a double-crust pie, so instead of separating the dough into two discs, leave it as one ball before refrigerating it.

Makes: One 9-by-13-inch pie (about 10 servings)

TOTAL SODIUM: 972 mg

SODIUM PER SERVING:
About 97 mg

---

1 recipe Pie Dough (page 73)

4 large eggs, divided

2 cups pumpkin puree

½ cup granulated sugar

½ cup firmly packed light brown sugar

2 teaspoons ground cinnamon

1 teaspoon ground ginger

¼ teaspoon ground allspice

¼ teaspoon light salt

⅛ teaspoon ground cloves

⅔ cup whole milk

⅔ cup heavy cream

1 tablespoon freshly squeezed lemon juice

1 teaspoon vanilla extract

1   Preheat the oven to 400 degrees F.

2   On a generously floured work surface, roll the dough out into a 12-by-16-inch rectangle about ⅛ inch thick. Gently fold the pastry in half and then in half again (but don't press down on it), so you can pick it up. Carefully transfer the pastry to a 9-by-13-inch baking sheet and unfold. Trim off the excess with scissors or a sharp knife so that the crust rises about ½ inch above the sides. Crimp the edges of the dough with your fingers or a fork. Reroll the scraps and use a cookie cutter or knife to cut out fun shapes. Place them on a separate baking sheet.

3   Make an egg wash: In a small bowl, using a fork, mix 1 of the eggs with 1 tablespoon of water. Brush the egg wash over the crimped edges of the dough and the dough cutouts. Cover the cutouts with plastic wrap, and refrigerate while you blind-bake the dough.

4   Cover the edges of the dough with aluminum foil, and line the bottom of the pastry with parchment paper. Top with pie weights or dried beans, and bake for 15 minutes, until lightly golden. Remove from the oven, remove the foil and parchment, and set aside.

5   Reduce the oven temperature to 350 degrees F.

6   In a blender or the bowl of a food processor (or in a large bowl using a wooden spoon), mix the pumpkin, both sugars, cinnamon, ginger, allspice, salt, and cloves until well combined, 1 to 2 minutes. Add the remaining 3 eggs, the milk, cream, lemon juice, and vanilla, and process until smooth, about 1 minute.

7   Pour the filling over the crust. Bake until the center is almost set, but still a little jiggly, 35 to 45 minutes. Remove the pie from the oven and set it on a wire rack to cool.

8   Bake the pastry shapes until light golden brown, about 10 minutes. Set them on another wire rack to cool. When they have cooled completely, arrange them decoratively on the pie.

Brown Butter Blondies

The key to a good blondie is to start with a tasty base, and browning the butter really elevates these. Then, of course, come the mix-ins. Adding unsalted toasted nuts is always a good choice, but you could also add chunks of dark or white chocolate, or dried fruit or citrus zest, or swirl some jam on the top before baking. I prefer these on the ooey-gooey side versus crisp, but they are good either way.

Makes: 9 blondies
TOTAL SODIUM: 341 mg
SODIUM PER BLONDIE:
About 38 mg

½ cup (1 stick) unsalted
  butter, cut into pieces

¾ cup lightly packed light
  brown sugar
1 tablespoon honey
1 cup (120 grams)
  all-purpose flour
½ teaspoon sodium-free
  baking powder

¼ teaspoon light salt
1 large egg
1 teaspoon vanilla extract
1 cup mix-ins, such as
  unsalted toasted nuts,
  chocolate chunks, or
  dried fruit

1   Preheat the oven to 325 degrees F. Line an 8-inch square pan with parchment paper.

2   In a medium, light-colored skillet, melt the butter over medium heat, and cook, stirring frequently, until the foam subsides, the butter is golden brown, and the solids have separated and turned a toasty brown, about 5 minutes. Stir in the brown sugar and honey. Transfer to a medium bowl, and set aside to cool slightly, at least 5 minutes.

3   In a small bowl, whisk together the flour, baking powder, and salt.

4   Whisk the egg and vanilla into the butter mixture until it turns creamy and light in color. Fold in the flour mixture, and then any mix-ins. Spoon the batter into the pan, smoothing the surface, and bake until just golden, 20 minutes for fudgier blondies or 25 for firmer ones. Cool for 10 minutes, then cut into 9 blondies.

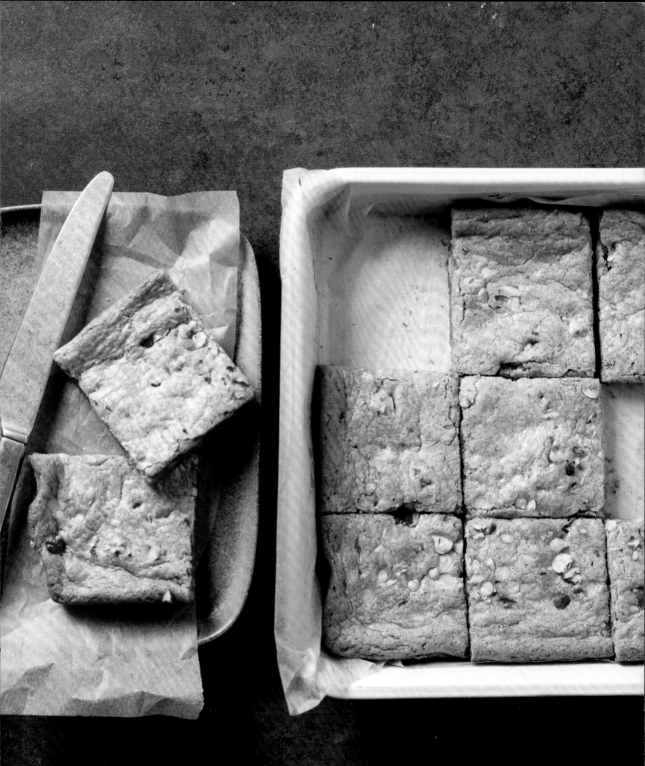

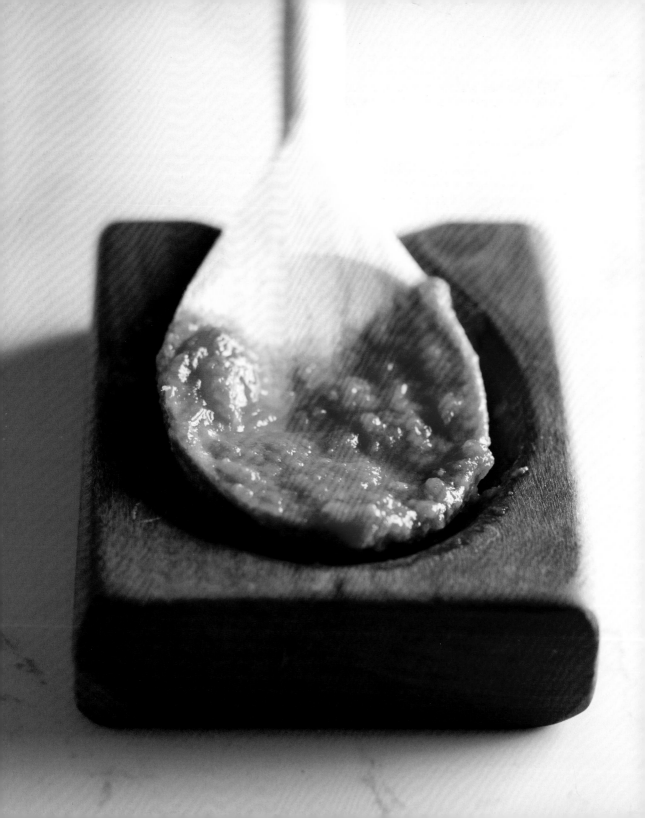

Acknowledgments

When I finished up my last book, on the heels of a diagnosis of Ménière's and a move to a low-sodium diet, I thought my cookbook-writing days were over. I have thought that before, but this time seemed different. How could I write a cookbook when I couldn't season recipes properly? So, I filed that world away as something that was fun while it lasted and moved on. And, perhaps unsurprisingly, almost immediately I started to write another cookbook. This time I had no intention of publishing it, however. I was writing it for myself. Writing down the recipes that made my life of low-sodium eating a joy.

I owe a big thank you to Susan Roxborough, Rachelle Longé McGhee, Tony Ong, and the crew at Sasquatch for helping me shape this book that I wrote "for me" into something that works for you.

I also would like to thank Dr. Jessica Shen for my diagnosis and the compassionate care. It's incredibly frustrating to have things going awry in your body and not know what is going on or what to do about it. Having the diagnosis and the treatment plan, while frustrating at first, has made a huge difference in my life. I've been almost entirely symptom free for over three years since adopting a low-sodium lifestyle.

Thanks to my fellow Ménière's folks on the Facebook Ménière's Disease Support Group. I might mostly be a lurker, but I've learned from your experiences and appreciate your feedback about which recipes interested you most.

To my "Family Dinner" friends, Hannah, Mike, Tori, Shelbi, Ross, and Molly—thank you all for your support by being mindful of sodium contents at our potlucks (not to mention gifting my books to all your friends and family!), especially in the early days.

Finally, a huge shout-out to my husband, Cameron, for adapting to the change in our daily diet (and putting up with me writing and shooting another cookbook—this time entirely in our house). It's one thing when you have to go low sodium for your own health, and another entirely when you are doing it for someone else. Thank you for your willingness to share in this adventure.

Sodium Counts for Common Ingredients

INGREDIENT	QUANTITY	SODIUM (MG)	SOURCE
BAKING			
Baking powder, sodium-free	1 teaspoon	0	Featherlight
Baking soda, sodium-free	1 teaspoon	0	Ener-G
Sugar, granulated or light brown	1 cup	0	365 Everyday
Corn syrup	1 tablespoon	15	Karo
Cornmeal, fine grind	1 cup	0	Bob's Red Mill
Cornstarch	1 ounce	0	365 Everyday
Honey	1 tablespoon	1	USDA
Maple syrup	1 tablespoon	0	365 Everyday
Wheat flour (all-purpose, bread, whole wheat, rye)	100 grams	2	USDA
Yeast, active dry	1 tablespoon	5	Bob's Red Mill
DAIRY			
Butter, unsalted	1 ounce	4	Plugra
Buttermilk	1 cup	216	Harrisburg dairy
Heavy cream	1 cup	80	Organic Valley
Milk, powdered	1 tablespoon	30	Giant
Milk, whole, 2%, or skim	1 cup	120	Horizon
Mozzarella, fresh	1 ounce	40	Whole Foods
Parmesan	1 ounce	180	Vivaldi
Sour cream	1 cup	120	Daisy Brand
Swiss cheese	1 ounce	44	365 Everyday
Yogurt, plain	1 cup	120	365 Organic
FRUITS			
Apples, quartered or chopped	1 cup	1	USDA
Blueberries	1 cup	1	USDA

INGREDIENT	QUANTITY	SODIUM (MG)	SOURCE
Honeydew, cubed	1 cup	32	USDA
Lemon juice	1 cup	2	USDA
Lime juice	1 cup	5	USDA
Mango, diced	1 cup	2	USDA
Peaches, slices	1 cup	0	USDA
Raspberries	1 cup	1	USDA

MEATS & SEAFOOD

INGREDIENT	QUANTITY	SODIUM (MG)	SOURCE
Beef, bones (such as short ribs)	1 pound	224	USDA
Beef, ground	1 pound	304	USDA
Beef, sirloin	1 pound	231	USDA
Chicken, skinless, boneless thighs (unbrined)	1 pound	432	USDA
Chicken, wings (unbrined)	1 pound	384	USDA
Egg yolk	1 large	14	USDA
Egg, whole	1 large	71	365 Everyday
Lamb, ground	1 pound	272	USDA
Pork, bone-in loin chops	1 pound	256	USDA
Pork, ground	1 pound	256	USDA
Pork, ribs or shoulder	1 pound	284	USDA
Salmon, fillet	1 pound	336	USDA
Tuna, canned, water-packed, no salt added	1 ounce	30	365 Everyday
Turkey, breast (unbrined)	1 pound	272	USDA

NUTS & GRAINS

INGREDIENT	QUANTITY	SODIUM (MG)	SOURCE
Almonds	1 cup	0	USDA
Barley, pearled	1 cup	18	USDA
Farro, semi-pearled	1 cup	0	365 Everyday
Oats, rolled or steel-cut	1 cup	0	365 Everyday
Pecans	1 cup	0	USDA
Rice, white long-grain	1 cup	9	USDA
Sesame seeds, whole	1 tablespoon	1	USDA
Tahini	1 cup	0	Nature's Pantry
Walnuts	1 cup	0	USDA

INGREDIENT	QUANTITY	SODIUM (MG)	SOURCE
SPICES & SEASONINGS			
Allspice, ground	1 teaspoon	1	USDA
Cayenne pepper, ground	1 tablespoon	2	USDA
Chilies, ancho or guaillo, dried	1 whole	7	USDA
Chilies, arbol, dried	1 whole	< 1	USDA
Cinnamon, ground	1 tablespoon	< 1	USDA
Coriander seeds, whole	1 tablespoon	2	USDA
Cumin, ground	1 tablespoon	10	USDA
Fennel seeds, whole	1 tablespoon	0	USDA
Garlic, dried powder	1 tablespoon	6	USDA
Mustard, whole seeds or dried powder	1 teaspoon	0	USDA
Nutmeg, ground	1 teaspoon	< 1	USDA
Onion, dried powder	1 tablespoon	5	USDA
Oregano, dried	1 tablespoon	1	USDA
Paprika, ground	1 tablespoon	5	USDA
Turmeric, ground	1 teaspoon	1	USDA
VEGETABLES & LEGUMES			
Arugula	1 cup	6	USDA
Asparagus	1 cup	3	USDA
Avocado, medium	1 whole	10	USDA
Beans, black, dried	1 cup	20	Camellia Brand
Beans, kidney, dried	1 cup	44	USDA
Beans, pinto, dried	1 cup	23	USDA
Beets, red, chopped	1 cup	106	USDA
Bell pepper, medium (red or yellow)	1 whole	4	USDA
Broccoli, chopped	1 cup	30	USDA
Carrots, chopped	1 cup	88	USDA
Cauliflower, chopped	1 cup	32	USDA
Celery, medium	1 stalk	32	USDA
Chickpeas, dried	1 cup	48	USDA
Cilantro, leaves	1 tablespoon	1	USDA
Corn, kernels	1 cup	23	USDA
Cucumber, medium	1 whole	4	USDA

INGREDIENT	QUANTITY	SODIUM (MG)	SOURCE
Dill	1 tablespoon	< 1	USDA
Eggplant, cubed	1 cup	2	USDA
Garlic	1 clove	< 1	USDA
Ginger, grated	1 tablespoon	< 1	USDA
Green chilies (Anaheim)	1 pound	16	USDA
Green onion, chopped	1 cup	16	USDA
Jalapeño, chopped	1 tablespoon	< 1	USDA
Kale, chopped	1 cup	11	USDA
Mint leaves	1 tablespoon	1	USDA
Mushrooms, crimini, sliced	1 cup	4	USDA
Onion, chopped	1 cup	6	USDA
Parsley, fresh flat-leaf	1 tablespoon	2	USDA
Peas, green	1 cup	7	USDA
Potatoes, fingerling	1 pound	16	USDA
Potatoes, Yukon Gold, medium	1 whole	12	USDA
Romaine, chopped	1 cup	8	USDA
Squash, winter, diced	1 cup	6	USDA
Sweet potatoes, cubed	1 cup	73	USDA
Thyme, fresh leaves	1 teaspoon	< 1	USDA
Tomato paste	1 ounce	5	Amore
Tomato puree	1 cup	20	Pomì
Tomato, cherry	1 whole	< 1	USDA
Tomato, canned chopped	1 cup	10	Pomì
Tomato, plum or slicing	1 pound	8	USDA

VINEGARS & OILS

Coconut aminos	1 teaspoon	90	Coconut Secret
Olive oil	1 tablespoon	0	365 Everyday
Vinegar, apple cider or distilled white	1 tablespoon	0	365 Everyday
Vinegar, balsamic	1 tablespoon	4	USDA
Vinegar, red wine	1 tablespoon	2	USDA
Vinegar, rice, unseasoned	1 tablespoon	0	Marukan

Index

Conversions

VOLUME

UNITED STATES	METRIC	IMPERIAL
¼ tsp.	1.25 mL	
½ tsp.	2.5 mL	
1 tsp.	5 mL	
½ Tbsp.	7.5 mL	
1 Tbsp.	15 mL	
⅛ c.	30 mL	1 fl. oz.
¼ c.	60 mL	2 fl. oz.
⅓ c.	80 mL	2.5 fl. oz.
½ c.	120 mL	4 fl. oz.
1 c.	230 mL	8 fl. oz.
2 c. (1 pt.)	460 mL	16 fl. oz.
1 qt.	1 L	32 fl. oz.

LENGTH

UNITED STATES	METRIC
⅛ in.	3 mm
¼ in.	6 mm
½ in.	1.25 cm
1 in.	2.5 cm
1 ft.	30 cm

WEIGHT

AVOIRDUPOIS	METRIC
¼ oz.	7 g
½ oz.	15 g
1 oz.	30 g
2 oz.	60 g
3 oz.	90 g
4 oz.	115 g
5 oz.	150 g
6 oz.	175 g
7 oz.	200 g
8 oz. (½ lb.)	225 g
9 oz.	250 g
10 oz.	300 g
11 oz.	325 g
12 oz.	350 g
13 oz.	375 g
14 oz.	400 g
15 oz.	425 g
16 oz. (1 lb.)	450 g
1½ lb.	750 g
2 lb.	900 g
2¼ lb.	1 kg
3 lb.	1.4 kg
4 lb.	1.8 kg

TEMPERATURE

OVEN MARK	FAHRENHEIT	CELSIUS	GAS
Very cool	250–275	120–135	½–1
Cool	300	150	2
Warm	325	165	3
Moderate	350	175	4
Moderately hot	375	190	5
Fairly hot	400	200	6
Hot	425	220	7
Very hot	450	230	8
Very hot	475	245	9

For ease of use, conversions have been rounded.

About the Author

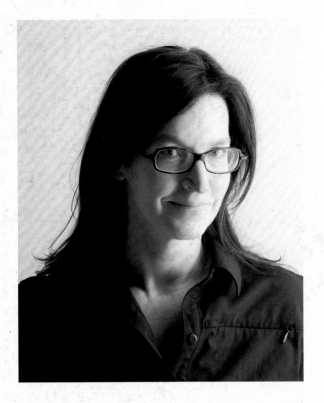

Lara Ferroni is a tech geek turned food geek who spends her days exploring and photographing food and cocktail culture. A writer and photographer, she is the author of six cookbooks, including *Doughnuts*, *An Avocado a Day*, *Real Snacks*, and *Put an Egg on It*. After being diagnosed with Ménière's disease, she found a whole new food project to master: low-sodium food that she actually wanted to eat. You can find more of her tasty photos and recipes on her blog, LaraFerroni.com.